The Yale

Steven B. Leder • Debra M. Suiter

The Yale Swallow Protocol

An Evidence-Based Approach to Decision Making

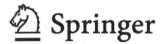 Springer

Steven B. Leder
Section of Otolaryngology
Department of Surgery
Yale School of Medicine
New Haven, CT, USA

Debra M. Suiter
VA Medical Center
Memphis, TN, USA

ISBN 978-3-319-05112-3   ISBN 978-3-319-05113-0 (eBook)
DOI 10.1007/978-3-319-05113-0
Springer Cham Heidelberg New York Dordrecht London

Library of Congress Control Number: 2014938105

Printed on acid-free paper

Springer is part of Springer Science+Business Media (www.springer.com)

Keep asking questions...You never know where the answers will lead.

Preface

We have made every effort to ensure that all information in this book is evidence-based and has been published in peer-reviewed journals. This is important in the area of swallow screening because many clinicians have their own idiosyncratic ways of doing things. And it works for them. Or does it? Without objective corroboration how do you know if your screening variables are reliable and providing facts versus what you want or think they are providing? How can you be sure that undefined tasks such as taking a sip of water or about a spoonful of pudding or a bite of a cracker are worthwhile without objective, and by this we mean instrumental, corroboration? Simply put you cannot. Without reliable confirmatory data all you are doing is wishful thinking and conjecture. It is important to remember that it is impossible to determine pharyngeal and laryngeal anatomy and physiology or bolus flow characteristics from clinical (bedside) observation. Since no one has X-ray vision the pharynx is a "black box" and whatever goes on in a black box is unknowable without direct observation.

Our analogy is: *Dysphagia goes with instrumental as aspiration risk goes with screening*. This was the impetus for development of the Yale Swallow Protocol. Questions you ask yourself as you read our book were asked by us as well. The answers are derived from rigorous research design and judicious interpretation of results. As you will see, we did not rely on a limited number of patients with homogeneous diagnoses. This would not have provided the generalizability desired in our screening test. Rather, over 5,000 patients from 14 different diagnostic categories and spanning the age spectrum from pediatric to geriatric participated in this programmatic line of research the culmination of which is the Yale Swallow Protocol.

You will find our methodology sound, the data supportive, and the recommendations beneficial. We trust that you will read and digest our new ideas with an open mind and then incorporate them into your daily clinical practice. This is reward enough for us. We are enormously privileged to participate in the care of our patients to the best of our abilities. And we wish the same for you.

New Haven, CT   Steven B. Leder
Memphis, TN   Debra M. Suiter

Acknowledgments

This book would not have been possible without the support and wisdom of our coauthors and colleagues. We gratefully acknowledge the expertise provided by Drs. Barry Green, Lewis Kaplan, David Karas, Joseph Murray, Alfred Rademaker, Mark Siegel, and Heather Warner; the insights provided by Mss. Lynn Acton, Karin Nystrom, Kelly Poskus, JoAnna Sloggy, and Brook Swainson; and the encouragement provided by Mr. Geoff Twohill. And we must thank our patients for the privilege of participating in their care as it is by them and for them that this programmatic line of research both began and will continue.

Contents

1 Building a Foundation and Defining Terms............ 1
Introduction... 2
Dysphagia Versus Aspiration Risk 2
Clinical or Bedside Swallow Examination Versus
Screening for Aspiration Risk 3
Why Screen with 3 Ounces Water? 5
Importance of a Swallowing Task 6
Laying the Research Foundation: Exponential
Increase of Swallowing Problems
in Geriatrics and the Frail Elderly 6
Introduction... 9
Statistical Underpinnings Necessary
to Understand What Constitutes a Good
Swallow Screen.. 15
References.. 15

**2 Screening Basics: Differentiating a Screen
from a Diagnostic Tool** 19
Introduction... 19
    Is Screening for Aspiration Risk Unique?............... 19
    Why Use a Screening Test to Determine
    Aspiration Risk? 22
    Accuracy of Screening Tests 23
Illustrative Example... 26
References.. 27

**3 Criteria Necessary for a Successful
and Reliable Swallow Screen** 29
Introduction... 29
What About Non-swallowing Stimuli? 31

Can Testing Be Done with Nasogastric
and Orogastric Feeding Tubes in Place? 32
What About Tracheotomy Tubes? 32
   Caveat Regarding the Yale Swallow Protocol
   and Tracheotomy Tube Use 32
Importance of Clinical Judgment 33
References 33

**4 Development of a Programmatic Line
of Research for Swallow Screening
for Aspiration Risk: The First Step** 35
Introduction 36
Three Research Questions 37
   Reliability Testing 40
Answers to the Three Research Questions 41
   3-Ounce Water Swallow Challenge and Liquid
   Aspiration Based on FEES Results 41
   3-Ounce Water Swallow Test and Diet
   Recommendations Based on FEES Results 42
   Synthesizing and Discussing the Results 46
Conclusions 47
References 48

**5 Development of a Protocol: Why You Need
More Than Just an Isolated 3-Ounce
Water Swallow Challenge** 51
Can a Brief Cognitive Examination Contribute
to the Assessment of Odds of Aspiration? 51
Introduction 53
Orientation Status 56
   Orientation: Thin Liquids 56
   Orientation: Puree 57
   Orientation: Oral Intake 58
Command Following 58
Command Following: Thin Liquids 59
   Command Following: Puree 59
   Command Following: Oral Intake 59
Clinical Importance 60

Can an Oral Mechanism Examination Contribute
to the Assessment of Odds of Aspiration? 62
Introduction 63
Reliability Testing 65
Labial Closure, Lingual Range of Motion,
Facial Symmetry, and Aspiration 66
References 69

6   **Generalizing the Yale Swallow**
    Protocol to Different Patient Populations:
    Time to Change 71
    Change Always Has Challenges but Challenges
    Can Only Be Overcome Through Change 72
    Generalization to the Pediatric Population 72
    Introduction 73
    Generalization to the Adult Acute Care Population 76
    Generalization to Trauma Patients 77
    Introduction 78
    Generalization to Stroke Patients 84
    Introduction 85
    Generalization to General Hospital Patients 88
    Introduction 89
    Overall Conclusions Based on the Four Studies:
    Pediatrics, Trauma, Acute Stroke,
    and General Hospital Populations 93
    References 95

7   **Recommending Specific Oral Diets Based**
    on Passing the Yale Swallow Protocol 99
    Introduction 99
    Importance of Ongoing Monitoring 101
    Tablet Swallowing 102
    References 103

8   **Yale Swallow Protocol Administration**
    and Interpretation: Passing and Failing 105
    Introduction 105
    Deferring Protocol Administration 106

Protocol Administration... 106
What to Do When the Protocol Is Passed 108
What to Do When the Yale Swallow
Protocol Is Failed... 108
References.. 109

9 **Implementation of the Yale Swallow
   Protocol by Other Health-Care Professionals**.......... 111
   Introduction.. 112
   References.. 117

10 **Question: What About Silent
    Aspiration? Answer: Silent Aspiration
    Is Volume-Dependent**.. 119
    Introduction.. 122
    References.. 128

11 **In Support of Use of the Yale
    Swallow Protocol: Longer-Term (5 Day)
    Success of Diet Recommendations
    and Oral Alimentation** 133
    Introduction.. 134
    Yale Swallow Protocol.. 135
    References.. 142

12 **Final Thoughts** 145
    Final Thoughts 146

13 **Yale Swallow Protocol Administration Forms**......... 149

Index... 153

Chapter 1
Building a Foundation and Defining Terms

Objectives: To discuss dysphagia versus aspiration risk, differences between the clinical or bedside examination versus a screening examination for aspiration risk, why use a 3-ounce water swallow challenge, and building a research foundation and rationale.

Methods: Definition of terms and geriatric population data sampling.

Results: Terms defined, justification for 3-ounce volume provided, and research foundation and rationale delineated.

Conclusions: All noninstrumental examinations can only determine probability of aspiration risk. A 3-ounce water swallow challenge is a swallow task that tests the limits of the swallowing system. The frail elderly geriatric population is growing exponentially and in order to provide state-of-the-art quality clinical care a reliable and validated swallow screen is required.

Keywords: Deglutition, Deglutition disorders, Swallow screening, Geriatrics, Oral alimentation

S.B. Leder and D.M. Suiter, *The Yale Swallow Protocol: An Evidence-Based Approach to Decision Making*, DOI 10.1007/978-3-319-05113-0_1, © Springer International Publishing Switzerland 2014

Introduction

Why write a book about swallow screening? Actually, it was for purely selfish reasons with a dose of self-preservation. The volume of new swallow consults had simply become too large to handle in our usual manner. Prior to 2008, all patients referred for a swallow test were evaluated instrumentally with either fiberoptic endoscopic evaluation of swallowing (FEES) [1, 2] or videofluoroscopic swallowing study (VFSS) [3]. We did this because we were unhappy with the state-of-the-evidence published on the accuracy and reliability of the clinical or bedside evaluation. The reported sensitivity and negative predictive values were too low and the false negative rates too high.

The consensus in the literature clearly showed that all clinical swallow screens were only 80–85 % accurate. In other words, there was the distinct possibility, nay we say certainty, that up to 20 % of referred patients would not be properly identified as having a swallow problem or, more precisely, be an aspiration risk, when, in fact, they were. This large percentage of false negatives was intolerable, not only for us but also for our referral base. Our professional referral base and patient consults would surely have dried up if one-fifth of referred patients were incorrectly identified as exhibiting no aspiration risk.

Dysphagia Versus Aspiration Risk

A distinction must be made between diagnosing dysphagia and determining potential aspiration risk. In order to diagnose dysphagia an instrumental evaluation, either FEES or VFSS, needs to be performed. Simply put, it is *impossible* to evaluate pharyngeal or laryngeal anatomy and physiology or bolus flow characteristics from a clinical examination. Why? The reason is the pharynx is akin to a "black box" when you as the clinician stand at the bedside and watch a patient swallow. As we often say, "You can see a lot by just looking," and that is precisely what one cannot do without the use of an instrumental assessment. Therefore, we will only be using the term *aspiration risk* when determining and discussing potential aspiration risk status with the Yale Swallow Protocol.

A swallowing screen is defined by the American Speech Language and Hearing Association (ASHA) as, "...a pass or fail procedure to identify individuals who require a comprehensive assessment of swallowing function or a referral for other professional and/or medical services" [4]. It is perfectly appropriate for a screening procedure to identify the presence or absence of a symptom which in this case is aspiration risk. If the procedure is being used to identify the abnormal anatomy and physiology causing the swallowing problem, i.e., dysphagia, then it is considered a diagnostic examination [5]. Therefore, the term diagnostic dysphagia evaluation will be reserved for procedures which define the anatomy and physiology of the swallow and can identify characteristics of bolus flow. Based on this definition, only instrumental measures, i.e., FEES or VFSS, are true diagnostic evaluations.

Clinical or Bedside Swallow Examination Versus Screening for Aspiration Risk

An important distinction that needs to be made involves the clinical or bedside Swallow examination (CSE). The criteria for a CSE versus screening for aspiration risk are not well defined in the literature, and it seems that it is left to the discretion of each individual clinician how they choose to classify their assessment of choice. Many clinicians use the term CSE to describe what is perceived to be a more thorough screening evaluation of swallowing, without using instrumental testing methods, by simply adding more subjective subsets and then integrating the combined information to reach a decision about swallowing success. Some clinicians even advocate for instituting interventions to improve the purported swallowing problems. But as discussed above, attempts at divining interventions to improve unknown pharyngeal and laryngeal anatomy and physiology and bolus flow characteristics are fraught with danger.

In general, a CSE may contain multiple assessment measures, e.g., a history component, a swallowing questionnaire, an oral mechanism evaluation, a brief cognitive assessment, and even oral feeding trials with various food consistencies and volumes, as well as therapeutic interventions or maneuvers, in an effort to understand and influence pharyngeal and laryngeal anatomy and physiology as well as bolus flow characteristics. Ironically, if one removed the CSE label it might be difficult to determine how clinicians classified their swallowing tool simply by looking at the assessment measures alone. However, it must be remembered that a CSE cannot identify anatomy, physiology, or bolus flow characteristics but rather only the presence or absence of aspiration risk.

Suiter and Leder [6] expanded on guidelines for swallow screening in clinical practice. We recognized the two aforementioned criteria for a screening test, i.e., to determine the likelihood of aspiration risk and to determine the need for further evaluation. A third important clinical criterion was that the screening tool had to be able to identify when and what type of oral alimentation to safely recommend. After all, this is what the referring physician wants to know, to wit, when it is appropriate to resume feeding the patient and what is the safest diet to recommend.

As will be discussed extensively, the Yale Swallow Protocol meets all criteria necessary to be a successful screening tool for determination of aspiration risk. It is simple and inexpensive to administer [7], quick to perform and interpret [8], reliable, accurate, and timely [9], validated for use with other health-care professionals (registered nurses) [10], applicable to virtually all patients regardless of diagnosis [6], and spanning the age spectrum from pediatric [11] to geriatric [6].

The protocol is strengthened by its key operating criteria and a unique factor not found in any other instrument. The key criteria include determination of aspiration risk with a sensitivity of 96.5 % [6], a negative predictive value of 97.9 % [6], and a false negative rate <2.0 % [12]. The unique factor is a priori knowledge of successful swallowing with thin liquid, puree, and, when appropriate, solid food consistencies because the 3-ounce challenge was performed in conjunction with and corroborated by both FEES [6] and VFSS [13]. This allows for specific oral diet recommendations to be made safely, confidently, and in a timely fashion without the need for instrumental dysphagia diagnostic testing [6] in virtually all hospitalized patients who are deemed potential candidates for oral alimentation [6, 14–16].

Why Screen with 3 Ounces Water?

Science is built upon a foundation that is made up of small steps and the foundation for the Yale Swallow Protocol is no different as it is based upon prior published research. There was no need for us to "reinvent the wheel" as it pertains to the components of the protocol. While a number of investigators have already used varying volumes of water as a component of a swallow screen, e.g., from 3 to 100 cc (30 cc = 1 ounce), none passed the accuracy threshold of ≥95 % correct identification of at-risk individuals [17] or incorporated research on odds of aspiration risk based on a brief cognitive assessment and an oral mechanism examination.

Fortunately, a study was available that, for us, used just the right volume for a water swallow challenge. There was no need to choose a unique volume for our research. DePippo et al. [18] investigated 44 stroke patients, who were in the rehabilitation, i.e., nonacute, setting, and used VFSS as the objective measure by which to validate their 3-ounce water swallow test. The patient was required to demonstrate uninterrupted drinking of 3 ounces of water without overt signs of aspiration. Failure criteria were inability to drink continuously, cough during or up to 1 min after completion of drinking, or a wet/hoarse voice quality post-swallow. The authors reported the relationship between cough and wet/hoarse voice quality on the screen and aspiration on VFSS to have a sensitivity of 76 % and a specificity of 59 %. Sensitivity and specificity of these same signs on the 3-ounce screen were revised to 94 and 26 % respectively when considering the relationship between these signs and aspiration of greater that 10 % of the bolus on VFSS. They went on to report that the relationship between these overt signs on the 3-ounce swallow and aspiration of thickened liquids or solids on VFSS was found to have a sensitivity of 94 % and a specificity of 30 %. A drawback of the study included a small and homogeneous sample population of only 44 stroke patients in the rehabilitation setting and a best-guess method regarding estimating the total volume of aspirated material, i.e., only scintigraphy can determine amount of aspirated material.

Importance of a Swallowing Task

We feel strongly that a screen must include a swallowing task and that task should "test the limits of the system." In other words, it should not be too easy to pass resulting in increased false negatives as well as not too hard to fail resulting in increased false positives. Very small bolus volumes or larger volumes but with sequential, i.e., interrupted, swallowing that mimicked small bolus volumes were to be avoided. Volumes >3 ounces were similarly to be avoided due to the potential that the majority of individuals would not normally drink this amount uninterrupted and, therefore, testing would not be transferrable to real-life situations. The 3-ounce volume has been shown to be ideal for this task. It was not too small making it too easy for patients to pass and thereby missing potential aspiration risk (false negatives). It was also not too large so as to be too hard for patients to perform successfully, thereby avoiding failing patients who were not aspiration risks (false positives). Chapter 2 provides the reader with necessary information on statistical measures that are needed for a reliable screening tool.

Laying the Research Foundation: Exponential Increase of Swallowing Problems in Geriatrics and the Frail Elderly

The original impetus for our work on swallow screening focused on the need for reliable determination of aspiration risk in the geriatric population [19]. Coinciding with our unease regarding use of currently published swallow screens was the growing knowledge that our target population is aging and aging rapidly. This is leading to disproportionately large numbers of the frail elderly being admitted to the hospital and concomitant with aging are many diagnoses having swallowing disorders and aspiration risk as a key symptom.

Dysphagia is a symptom and although aging, per se, does not cause dysphagia the potential for development of swallowing disorders becomes increasingly more common with advancing age [20–26]. The well elderly retain adequate functional reserve to compensate for the normal slowing of physiologic swallowing parameters, but when stress intervenes, e.g., due to illness, trauma, surgery, or declining neurological status, functional reserve may fall below the level required for successful maintenance of activities of daily living including, importantly, oral alimentation [27, 28].

Population projections indicate that between 2000 and 2030 the number of individuals 65 years and older will more than double, from 35 to 72 million, i.e., increasing from 12 to nearly 20 % of the U.S. population; and old old individuals 85+ years will comprise 25 % of this older population by 2060 [29]. Given the potential for increased morbidity and mortality associated with swallowing problems in the elderly hospitalized patient [22, 23], it is important to understand trends in dysphagia referral rates and determine optimal swallow screening to provide appropriate, timely, and safe determination of both aspiration risk and oral diet recommendations.

We present here the only long-term, large, longitudinal, epidemiological study which investigated referral rates, sex, age, diagnostic categories, and incidence of dysphagia and aspiration risk status in a referred sample of hospitalized patients [19]. The purpose of this investigation was to describe the epidemiology and changing demographic trends relative to aging and referrals for swallowing testing in the acute care setting with an emphasis on the elderly hospitalized population and use of the Yale Swallow Protocol as a valid, reliable, and patient friendly screening tool to use for determination of aspiration risk and diet recommendations.

Leder SB, Suiter DM. An epidemiologic study on aging and dysphagia in the acute care hospitalized population: 2000–2007. Gerontology. 2009;55:714–8.

(Used and modified with permission from S. Karger AG, Basel.)

Objectives: To describe total and yearly demographic trends relative to aging, dysphagia referral rates, and oral feeding status in hospitalized patients from 2000 through 2007.

Methods: A prospective, consecutive, referred sample of 4,038 hospitalized patients from a large, urban, tertiary, acute care, teaching hospital participated. Dysphagia referral rates were described according to year, age (decade), sex, admitting diagnostic category, results of dysphagia evaluations, and oral feeding status. Diagnosis of dysphagia and feeding status made objectively with FEES.

Results: Dysphagia referral rates doubled between 2000 and 2007, with increases of 20 % per year and increases in all decades from 2002 through 2007. Over 70 % of dysphagia referrals were for older patients 60+ years and over 42 % of these were old old patients 80+ years. Referrals for 80–89 year old old patients almost doubled and 90+ year old old patients more than tripled between 2000 and 2007. In older patients 60+ years, 62.3 % (1,771/2,843) did not exhibit dysphagia, 18.0 % (513/2,843) benefited from specific diet modifications to reduce aspiration risk, and 19.7 % (559/2,843) were made nil-by-mouth due to severe dysphagia and aspiration.

Conclusions: From 2000 to 2007, dysphagia referrals across all ages increased 20 %/year, with more referrals for older (70.4 %) than younger patients (29.6 %), and the old old patient referrals doubling to tripling. To reestablish oral alimentation and hydration as soon as possible following a dysphagia referral in this medically fragile population, an evidence-based screening tool to determine potential aspiration risk, i.e., the Yale Swallow Protocol, is recommended. The protocol includes a brief cognitive assessment, oral mechanism evaluation, and a 3-ounce water swallow challenge with progression to FEES or VFSS testing only if failed.

Keywords: Deglutition, Deglutition disorders, Geriatrics, Swallow screening, Fiberoptic endoscopy, Oral alimentation

Introduction

Between January 01, 2000 and December 31, 2007 a prospective, consecutive, referred sample of 4,038 inpatients from the acute care setting of a large urban tertiary care teaching hospital were evaluated objectively with FEES. Participant demographics (Table 1.1) and admitting diagnostic categories grouped by age, i.e., younger 0–59 years versus older patients 60–90+ years (Table 1.2), are presented. Old patients were defined as between 60 and 79 years of age and old old patients were defined as 80+ years of age. All patients were tested with FEES and given the 3-ounce water swallow challenge. We were thereby able to determine dysphagia, aspiration status, and diet recommendations with instrumental testing and correlate these data with aspiration risk as determined by the Yale Swallow Protocol.

In the younger age group (0–59 years), the two most common admitting diagnostic categories were medical (26.9 %; 320/1,191) and neurological (19.6 %; 233/1,191) (Table 1.2). In this group, 69.3 % (828/1,195) of patients did not exhibit dysphagia, but 30.7 % (367/1,195) did exhibit dysphagia. Of these patients with dysphagia, 51.5 % (189/367) benefited from specific diet modifications to reduce aspiration risk while 48.5 % (178/367) were made nil-by-mouth due to severe dysphagia and aspiration.

TABLE 1.1. Participant demographic information (Used with permission from S. Karger AG, Basel: Leder SB, Suiter DM. An epidemiologic study on aging and dysphagia in the acute care hospitalized population: 2000–2007. Gerontology. 2009:55:714–8.)

			Ages 0–59	Ages 60–105
Gender	Males	N	743 (62.3 %)	1,538[a] (54.2 %)
	Females	N	450 (37.5 %)	1,302 (45.8 %)
Mean age	Males	$\bar{X}$	45.2 years	76.4 years
		Range	2.2–59.0 years	60.0–105.0 years
	Females	$\bar{X}$	45.6 years	78.9 years
		Range	2.2–59.0 years	60.0–105.0 years

[a]Missing data for 5 (.3 %) participants

TABLE 1.2.   Participant admitting diagnostic categories by age (Used with permission from S. Karger AG, Basel: Leder SB, Suiter DM. An epidemiologic study on aging and dysphagia in the acute care hospitalized population: 2000–2007. Gerontology. 2009:55:714–8.)

Diagnostic category	Number of participants	
	Age 0–59 years	Age 60–105 years
Cardiothoracic surgery	34 (2.9 %)	180 (6.4 %)
Esophageal surgery	30 (2.5 %)	47 (1.7 %)
Head and neck surgery	61 (5.1 %)	110 (3.9 %)
Neurosurgery	163 (13.7 %)	152 (5.4 %)
Medical	320 (26.9 %)	877 (30.9 %)
Pulmonary	144 (12.0 %)	490 (17.3 %)
Cancer	58 (4.9 %)	109 (3.9 %)
Left stroke	59 (4.9 %)	240 (8.5 %)
Right stroke	58 (4.9 %)	199 (7.0 %)
Brain stem stroke	22 (1.8 %)	32 (1.1 %)
Parkinson's disease	7 (.6 %)	23 (.8 %)
Dementia	2 (.2 %)	123 (4.3 %)
Traumatic brain injury or other neurological	233 (19.6 %)	249 (8.8 %)
Total	1,191[a]	2,831[b]

[a]Missing data for 4 (.3 %) participants

[b]Missing data for 12 (.4 %) participants

In the older age group (60+ years), the two most common admitting diagnostic categories were general medical (30.9 %; 877/2,831) and pulmonary (17.3 %; 490/2,831) (Table 1.2). In this group, 62.3 % (1,771/2,843) of participants did not exhibit dysphagia, but 37.7 % (1,072/2,843) did exhibit dysphagia. Of these patients with dysphagia, 47.9 % (513/1,072) benefited from specific diet modifications to reduce aspiration risk while 52.1 % (559/1,072) were made nil-by-mouth due to severe dysphagia and aspiration.

Table 1.3 shows cross tabulation epidemiologic data by age (decade), test year, and totals. Referral rates for dysphagia testing increased approximately 20 % per year from 2002 to 2007 and doubled between 2000 and 2007, resulting in an increased number of participants in all age decades from 2002 through 2007. The actual number of the 80–89 year old old referrals almost doubled

TABLE 1.3.   Population data for age by test year (Used with permission from S. Karger AG, Basel: Leder SB, Suiter DM. An epidemiologic study on aging and dysphagia in the acute care hospitalized population: 2000–2007. Gerontology. 2009:55:714–8.)

Decade		Test year								
		2000	2001	2002	2003	2004	2005	2006	2007	Total
1	N	6	2	3	9	8	12	15	11	66
	%	1.4	.5	.9	2.3	1.7	2.2	2.3	1.3	1.6
2	N	12	6	7	10	11	13	17	31	107
	%	2.8	1.6	2.1	2.6	2.4	2.4	2.6	3.6	2.6
3	N	17	17	12	17	13	18	19	22	135
	%	4.0	4.6	3.6	4.3	2.8	3.3	2.9	2.6	3.3
4	N	39	20	28	35	33	54	54	65	328
	%	9.1	5.4	8.5	9.0	7.1	9.9	8.2	7.6	8.1
5	N	56	55	36	33	74	68	96	141	559
	%	13.1	14.9	10.9	8.4	16.0	12.5	14.6	16.4	13.8
6	N	68	53	48	65	73	95	124	161	687
	%	15.9	14.4	14.5	16.6	15.8	17.5	18.9	18.8	17.0
7	N	113	99	86	95	121	115	145	182	956
	%	26.4	26.8	26.1	24.3	26.2	21.1	22.1	21.2	23.7
8	N	98	93	88	104	100	121	142	185	931
	%	22.9	25.2	26.7	26.6	21.6	22.2	21.6	21.6	23.1
9	N	19	24	22	23	29	48	44	60	269
	%	4.4	6.5	6.7	5.9	6.3	8.8	6.7	7.0	6.7
Total		428	369	330	391	462	544	656	858	4,038

and the 90+ year old old referrals more than tripled between 2000 and 2007. The 80–90+ year old old referrals comprised 42.2 % (1,200/2,843) of the total older population sample. In addition, there were more total referrals for the older group between 60 and 90+ years, i.e., 70.4 % (2,843/4,038), versus the younger group between 0 and 59 years, i.e., 29.6 % (1,195/4,038).

Table 1.4 shows oral feeding status by decade by sex distribution. Referrals for male patients both increased in every decade and outnumbered female referrals through decade 7. But this trend changed to more referrals for females and females outnumbered male referrals in decades 8 and 9. Females swallowed significantly more successfully than males for decade 6 (N=686; X^2=8.019; $p \le .005$), decade 7 (N=954; X^2=5.611; $p<.019$), and decade 8 (N=929; X^2=22.158; $p<.001$).

TABLE 1.4.   Oral feeding status by decade by sex (Used with permission from S. Karger AG, Basel: Leder SB, Suiter DM. An epidemiologic study on aging and dysphagia in the acute care hospitalized population: 2000–2007. Gerontology. 2009:55:714–8.)

Decade											
Sex		1	2	3	4	5	6*	7*	8*	9	Total**
Male											
PO[a]	N	36	71	73	159	282	330	415	336	90	1,792
	%	92.3	92.2	86.9	83.2	80.1	77.3	76.9	73.7	78.3	78.6
NPO[b]	N	3	6	11	32	70	97	125	120	25	489
	%	7.7	7.8	13.1	16.8	19.9	22.7	23.1	26.3	21.7	21.4
Total		39	77	84	191	352	427	540	456	115	2,281
Female											
PO	N	25	26	47	120	175	223	344	407	134	1,501
	%	92.6	89.7	92.2	87.6	85.4	86.1	83.1	86.0	87.0	85.8
NPO	N	2	3	4	17	30	36	70	66	20	248
	%	7.4	10.3	7.8	12.4	14.6	13.9	16.9	14.0	13.0	14.2
Total		27	2	51	137	205	259	414	473	154	1,749

*Significantly more females than males were able to tolerate an oral diet for decade 6 ($N=686$; $X^2=8.019$; $p \leq .005$), decade 7 ($N=954$; $X^2=5.611$; $p<.019$), and decade 8 ($N=929$; $X^2=22.158$; $p<.001$)

**Data are missing for 8 (.2 %) of patients

[a]PO=by mouth

[b]NPO=nil-by-mouth

Referrals for dysphagia testing almost doubled for 80–89 year old old patients and more than tripled for 90+ year old old patients between 2000 and 2007. This is consistent with U.S. population projections for 2060 [29]. In addition, 70 % of total referrals were for 60–90+ year older patients, with 42 % of these referrals for 80–90+ year old old patients. There are three interrelated reasons for the observed increase in referral rates for dysphagia testing across all age decades and for older patients in particular. First, an aging population results in increased hospital admissions resulting in a larger pool of potential patients for dysphagia referrals. Second, there is enhanced physician awareness of the need for evidence-based dysphagia testing. Third, the dysphagia specialist is providing useful patient care information which generates more dysphagia referrals, i.e., the Yale Swallow Protocol is performing as it should be.

Not all referrals for suspected dysphagia and aspiration risk result in a positive finding. In fact, over 60 % of referrals in both the younger and older age groups were negative allowing for immediate resumption of oral alimentation, hydration, and medications. It is important, therefore, to evaluate the patient as soon as possible so as not to delay reestablishment of eating and drinking. A recent series of studies have been published to achieve this goal. The protocol starts with a brief cognitive screen to determine if cognitive abilities are adequate to participate safely in the protocol [30], completion of an oral mechanism examination [31], and passing the 3-ounce water swallow challenge [6].

It is important to note that results of the brief cognitive screen [30] and oral mechanism examination [31] provide the clinician information only on odds of aspiration risk when performing the 3-ounce water swallow challenge and should not necessarily be used as exclusionary criteria for screening. That is, some patients will pass the 3-ounce challenge despite some degree of altered mental status and impaired oral mechanism functioning.

If the protocol is failed, objective testing with FEES or VFSS is performed. FEES is especially well suited for use in the older patient population as it is done at bedside allowing for family members to be present and with no time limit due to avoidance of irradiation exposure; is safe, repeatable, patient-friendly, and uses regular food; and is easily scheduled and can be performed independently by a speech-language pathologist [32]. In addition, both diet modifications, e.g., bolus consistency changes with thickened liquids and bolus volume changes, as well as swallowing strategies, e.g., effortful swallow, swallow-clear throat-swallow again, and two swallows/bolus, can be tried during FEES and VFSS to determine objectively their success in promoting safe swallowing.

If non-oral feeding is recommended the patient should be reassessed for candidacy for a swallow reevaluation within a few days since rapid improvement in medical condition or cognitive status often occurs in the acute care setting [32]. Specifically, the Yale Swallow Protocol, which includes the 3-ounce water swallow challenge, is repeated and, if passed, an oral diet can be recommended. If failed again, further instrumental testing may be indicated. Serial FEES evaluations have been shown to be effective in determining when best to resume successful oral feeding and what bolus consistencies to use for optimal swallowing success [32].

There were more dysphagia referrals for males, both total and through decade 7, but then more dysphagia referrals for females in decades 8 and 9 (Table 1.4). This is consistent with gender projections for the U.S. population through 2060 [29]. There were significant differences in the incidence of dysphagia in males versus females dependent upon age decade. In addition, males may be hospitalized more frequently than females, leading to increased dysphagia referrals. An increase in female referrals for dysphagia testing in the old old 80+ year group is attributed to longer female life expectancy.

The increase in aging of the general population [29], combined with the present study's observed increase in dysphagia referrals for older patients, will result in increased demand for dysphagia testing at least through 2060 and probably longer. This will require, in addition to speech-language pathologists, a more diverse set of health-care professionals and clinicians who are trained to screen for aspiration risk. For example, both registered and advanced-practice nurses, as well as physicians and other independent licensed practitioners such as physician assistants, can and should screen for aspiration risk. This holds true for both acute care and rehabilitative environments. It is imperative, however, that appropriate evidence-based swallow screening tools be used and followed, when necessary, by instrumental diagnostic techniques. This will prevent unnecessary morbidity associated with dysphagia and aspiration risk in the geriatric population and promote safe oral alimentation for optimal health and quality-of-life enhancement [20].

Conclusions

In conclusion, during an 8-year study period, from 2000 to 2007, dysphagia referrals across all ages increased 20 %/year, with more referrals for older (70.4 %) than younger patients (29.6 %), and with the old old patient referrals doubling to tripling in number. Since older adults are the fastest growing age group in the United States it is expected that incidence of swallowing disorders and aspiration risk will increase commensurately as the older population more than doubles by 2060. Increases of this magnitude make it imperative that evidence-based screening tests for aspiration risk be established and implemented by trained professionals.

Therefore, in order to promote safe resumption of oral alimentation, hydration, and medications as soon as possible following a referral for swallow testing in this medically fragile population, an evidence-based screening protocol, i.e., the Yale Swallow Protocol, is recommended that incorporates a brief cognitive assessment [30], an oral mechanism examination [31], and a 3-ounce water swallow challenge [6] with progression to instrumental testing with FEES or VFSS only if the protocol is failed [10].

Statistical Underpinnings Necessary to Understand What Constitutes a Good Swallow Screen

Based on the foundation provided by the geriatric data one can grasp the importance of being able to use a reliable, validated, and generalizable swallow screen to determine potential aspiration risk prior to beginning oral alimentation. Similarly, it is vital to understand the statistical terms and criteria on which a good swallow screen is based. A working knowledge of the statistics relevant to the general topic area of screening tests enables and enhances a clinician's ability to evaluate a given screen's strengths and weaknesses. The goal is to allow for an educated decision to be made when choosing a screen to use for the important decision of determining a patient's potential aspiration risk and oral feeding status. Chapter 2 provides this information.

References

1. Langmore SE, Schatz MA, Olsen N. Fiberoptic endoscopic examination of swallowing safety: a new procedure. Dysphagia. 1988; 2:216–9.
2. Langmore SE, Schatz MA, Olsen N. Endoscopic and videofluoroscopic evaluations of swallowing and aspiration. Ann Otol Rhinol Laryngol. 1991;100:678–81.

3. Logemann JA. Evaluation and treatment of swallowing disorders. 2nd ed. Austin, TX: Pro-Ed; 1998.

4. American Speech-Language-Hearing Association. Preferred practice patterns for the profession of speech-language pathology [Preferred practice patterns]. www.asha.org/policy.

5. Logeman JA, Veiss S, Colangelo L. A screening procedure for oropharyngeal dysphagia. Dysphagia. 1999;14:44–51.

6. Suiter DM, Leder SB. Clinical utility of the 3 ounce water swallow test. Dysphagia. 2008;23:244–50.

7. Heffner JE. Swallowing complications after endotracheal extubation. Chest. 2010;137:509–10.

8. Cochrane AL, Holland WW. Validation of screening procedures. Br Med Bull. 1971;27:3–8.

9. Kertscher B, Speyer R, Palmieri M, Plant C. Bedside screening to detect Oropharyngeal dysphagia in patients with neurological disorders: an updated systematic review. Dysphagia. 2014;29:204–12.

10. Warner HL, Suiter DM, Nystrom K, Poskus, K, Leder SB. Comparing accuracy of the 3-ounce water swallow challenge dysphagia screening protocol when administered by registered nurses and speech-language pathologists. J Clin Nurs. (In Press). doi:10.1111/jocn.12340.

11. Suiter DM, Leder SB, Karas DE. The 3-ounce (90 cc) water swallow challenge: a screening test for children with suspected oropharyngeal dysphagia. Otolaryngol Head Neck Surg. 2009;140:187–90.

12. Leder SB, Suiter DM, Green BG. Silent aspiration risk is volume dependent. Dysphagia. 2011;26:304–9.

13. Suiter DM, Sloggy J, Leder SB. Validation of the Yale Swallow Protocol: a prospective double-blinded videofluoroscopic study. Dysphagia. 2014;29:199–203.

14. Leder SB, Suiter DM, Warner HL, Kaplan LJ. Initiating safe oral feeding in critically ill intensive care and step-down unit patients based on passing a 3-ounce (90 milliliters) water swallow challenge. J Trauma. 2011;70:1203–7.

15. Leder SB, Suiter DM, Warner HL, Acton LM, Swainson BA. Success of recommending oral diets in acute stroke patients based on a 90-cc water swallow challenge protocol. Top Stroke Rehabil. 2012;19:40–4.

16. Leder SB, Suiter DM, Warner HL, Acton LM, Siegel MD. Safe initiation of oral diets in hospitalized patients based on passing a 3-ounce (90 cc) water swallow challenge protocol. Q J Med. 2012;105:257–63.

17. Leder SB, Espinosa JF. Aspiration risk after acute stroke: comparison of clinical examination and fiberoptic endoscopic evaluation of swallowing. Dysphagia. 2002;17:214–8.

18. DePippo KL, Holas MA, Reding MJ. Validation of the 3-oz water swallow test for aspiration following stroke. Arch Neurol. 1992; 49:1259–61.

19. Leder SB, Suiter DM. An epidemiologic study on aging and dysphagia in the acute care hospitalized population: 2000–2007. Gerontology. 2009;55:714–8.

20. Sheth N, Diner WC. Swallowing problems in the elderly. Dysphagia. 1988;2:209–15.
21. Robbins J, Hamilton JW, Lof GL, Kempster GB. Oropharyngeal swallowing in normal adults of different ages. Gastroenterology. 1992; 103:823–9.
22. Schindler JS, Kelly JH. Swallowing disorders in the elderly. Laryngoscope. 2002;112:589–602.
23. Marik PE, Kaplan D. Aspiration pneumonia and dysphagia in the elderly. Chest. 2003;124:328–36.
24. Leslie P, Drinnan MJ, Ford GA, Wilson JA. Swallow respiratory patterns and aging: presbyphagia or dysphagia? J Gerontol. 2005;60A:391–5.
25. McCullough GH, Rosenbek JC, Wertz RT. Defining swallowing function by age. Top Geriatr Rehabil. 2007;23:290–307.
26. Roy N, Stemple J, Merrill RM, Thomas L. Dysphagia in the elderly: preliminary evidence of prevalence, risk factors, and socioemotional effects. Ann Otol Rhinol Laryngol. 2007;116:858–65.
27. Pendergast DR, Fisher NM, Calkins E. Cardiovascular, neuromuscular, and metabolic alterations with age leading to frailty. J Gerontol. 1993;48:61–7.
28. Leder SB. Incidence and type of aspiration in acute care patients requiring mechanical ventilation via a new tracheotomy. Chest. 2002; 122:1721–6.
29. U.S. Census Projections. Projections of the population by selected age groups and sex for the United States: 2015 to 2060. www.census.gov
30. Leder SB, Suiter DM, Warner HL. Answering orientation questions and following single step verbal commands: effect on aspiration status. Dysphagia. 2009;24:290–5.
31. Leder SB, Suiter DM, Murray J, Rademaker AW. Can an oral mechanism examination contribute to the assessment of odds of aspiration? Dysphagia. 2013;28:370–4.
32. Leder SB. Serial fiberoptic endoscopic swallowing evaluations in the management of patients with dysphagia. Arch Phys Med Rehabil. 1998;79:1264–9.

Chapter 2
Screening Basics: Differentiating a Screen from a Diagnostic Tool

Objectives: To provide knowledge and understanding regarding differentiating a screen from a diagnostic tool and why a reliable and validated swallow screen is valuable for patient care.

Methods: Definition of statistical terms necessary for understanding the bases for swallow screening.

Results: Terms defined were sensitivity, specificity, positive predictive value, negative predictive value, positive likelihood ratio, negative likelihood ratio, false positive rates, and false negative rates.

Conclusions: Understanding the statistical underpinnings pertinent to swallow screening will provide the clinician with the knowledge necessary to make informed decisions regarding use of the best swallow screen for patient care.

Keywords: Deglutition, Deglutition disorders, Swallow screening, Statistics, Oral alimentation

Introduction

Is Screening for Aspiration Risk Unique?

The direct and accurate answer is No. Dysphagia specialists like to think that screening tests for aspiration risk are different from, for example, screening tests for pregnancy, high blood pressure, tuberculosis, or diabetes but screening for aspiration risk is no different from screening for any other potential symptom, condition, or disease that is screened for in medicine. What is critically important, however, is use of a validated, reliable, and generalizable screen that can be used for the vast majority of at-risk individuals. You must then trust the screen to do its job and abide by its results. If this is not the case, then the screen is useless and you must test all referred individuals with the more expensive, time-consuming, and personnel-laden instrumental evaluation which in the case of dysphagia is either an endoscopic or videofluoroscopic procedure.

In order to be beneficial, a screening test must be easy to administer, accurate, and require less time, expense, and staff resources than a diagnostic test. In medicine, screening tests are generally given to groups of asymptomatic people to detect potential disease indicators. Groups can range from the population as a whole to more individualized, case-finding approaches focusing on individuals at-risk for a specific target condition [1]. Conversely, the purpose of a diagnostic test is to confirm the presence or absence of the target condition. A screening test, therefore, will have high sensitivity but low specificity, thereby allowing detection of most patients with the target condition while having the acceptable disadvantage of a high false positive rate. Subsequent diagnostic testing will eliminate the over-referrals, i.e., false positives, from receiving treatment.

A screen has both different goals and different endpoints than a diagnostic evaluation. A screen is a simple, noninvasive, and inexpensive method of detecting the probability that an individual has a disease. For the purposes of this book just substitute aspiration risk for disease. A screen cannot and does not provide a definitive diagnosis. Typically, screening tests are given to large groups of asymptomatic people, whereas diagnostic tests are given either to symptomatic individuals to establish a diagnosis or to asymptomatic individuals who fail a screening.

In clinical practice, it is neither practical nor feasible to screen everyone. Therefore, it is customary for a screening test to adopt a more individualized or case-finding approach [1]. In case-finding, individuals who are considered to be at high risk for a particular condition are tested. For instance, it is common knowledge that health-care workers are considered to be at higher risk than the general population for exposure to tuberculosis and, therefore, receive an annual screening test for that disease. Other examples of screening tests that use a case-finding approach include mammograms for women over age 40 years and colonoscopies for individuals over age 50 years. *It is important to note that when a screening test is passed no further treatment or assessment is indicated.* Only when a screening test is failed is the more extensive and expensive diagnostic examination performed.

The use of a screening test is based upon two general assumptions [1]. First, the course of the targeted disorder will, if undetected and untreated, result in serious and preventable health problems. For example, undetected prandial aspiration has the potential to cause a number of negative health outcomes including aspiration pneumonia, acute respiratory failure, dehydration, malnutrition, and sepsis with the possibility of leading to death. Therefore, early identification and management is essential in prevention and health maintenance. Second, treatment for the target condition being screened exists and is effective. Again, in the case of prandial aspiration, effective interventions such as postural changes, bolus volume adjustments, and viscosity alterations can be implemented with the goal of either eliminating or minimizing its consequences. A nil per os, i.e., no food or drink by mouth, order is generally effective when prandial aspiration is unresolved and before instrumental testing is performed.

A screening test yields a binary response. A positive result, i.e., pass, indicates that further testing is necessary to determine if the disease or condition being screened for is truly present. A negative result, i.e., fails, indicates that the individual most likely does not have the disease or condition being screened for and further testing is not necessary. Specific to swallow screening, the binary pass or fail determination will identify an individual who either is in no need of additional testing and is not an aspiration risk or requires further diagnostic assessment to confirm a swallowing disorder. A diagnostic swallowing test is not a pass or fail procedure. Rather, the purpose is to identify the underlying pathophysiology of the swallowing disorder that results in signs or symptoms of dysphagia and then to determine an appropriate treatment to address this pathophysiology with the goal of promoting safe and successful swallowing.

Why Use a Screening Test to Determine Aspiration Risk?

Despite the fact that pulmonary aspiration remains a leading cause of nosocomial infection in the critically ill [2], it is neither medically necessary nor fiscally defensible to perform instrumental swallow testing on all patients referred for swallowing testing. It is, however, vitally important to have a plan with the goal of identifying those specific patients who may have a high aspiration risk prior to initiating oral alimentation and medications.

All patients deemed to have potential swallowing problems should be screened for aspiration risk. The goal is to administer a reliable swallowing screen to all appropriately identified patients, deemed appropriate to begin oral alimentation, before starting oral ingestion of foods, fluids, or medications. This is especially important as many patients have an a priori increased aspiration risk due to comorbidities and concomitant interventions including short- (<24 h) [3] or longer-term (>24 h) endotracheal intubation [4–6], traumatic brain injury [5], other cognitive issues [7], severe deconditioning and reduced functional reserve [8], medication side effects [8], and advanced age [9, 10].

The use of screening tools to identify patients with potential aspiration risk has garnered substantial interest from a number of health-care organizations, including the American Heart Association, the Veterans Health Administration, and the American Speech-Language-Hearing Association, who recognize the need for early identification and appropriate intervention for identified individuals. Use of screening tests to detect aspiration risk is supported in that hospitals which used a mandatory and formal swallow screening procedure reported lower rates of pneumonia, and concomitant cost savings than those without [11–13].

Accuracy of Screening Tests

In order to determine accuracy of a screening tool, a 2×2 contingency table is frequently used. Such a table allows for results of the screening tool to be compared to those of a reference standard test. Results are classified as either positive or negative and the criterion for each of these is set a priori. Table 2.1 shows a typical 2×2 table which includes:

1. The number of true positives or those individuals that have the disease and test positive.
2. The number of false positives or those individuals that do not have the disease and test positive.
3. The number of false negatives or those individuals that do have the disease and test negative.
4. The number of true negatives or those individuals that do not have the disease and test negative.

Both true and false positives and negatives are used to calculate the statistical measures of sensitivity, specificity, positive predictive value (PPV), and negative predictive value (NPV). These measures provide information about the validity of a test. The accuracy of a screening test is generally expressed in terms of its sensitivity and specificity. A high sensitivity, therefore, is good.

TABLE 2.1.   A typical 2×2 contingency table.

| | | Reference standard (FEES or VFSS) | |
		Positive	Negative
Screening	Positive	a or True Positives (TP)	b or False Positives (FP)
	Negative	c or False Negatives (FN)	d or True Negatives (TN)

Sensitivity $= a/(a+c)$
Specificity $= d/(b+d)$
PPV $= a/(a+b)$
NPV $= d/(c+d)$
Positive Likelihood Ratio $=$ Sensitivity$/(1-$Specificity$)$
Negative Likelihood Ratio $= (1-$Sensitivity$)/$Specificity

On the other hand, low specificity, i.e., a low false negative rate, is an inherent shortcoming for all screening tests so as not to miss people who actually have the target condition. Similarly, an acceptable disadvantage of a screening test is a high rate of false positives, which means that screening tests often over-refer individuals for full diagnostic testing. Ideally, a reliable and clinically useful screen for aspiration risk should have a high sensitivity, a high negative predictive value, and a low false negative rate.

In contrast, diagnostic or criterion standard tests should have high sensitivity in order to identify people who truly have the target condition as well as high specificity in order to eliminate people who truly do not have the target condition. It must be remembered that the goal of a diagnostic tests is to make a definitive diagnosis.

Sensitivity

Sensitivity of a test is the proportion of individuals with the target condition who have a positive test result. In other words, sensitivity measures a test's ability to identify an individual with the disease as positive. Tests that are found to be highly sensitive indicate that there are few false negative results and thus fewer cases of disease are missed [14]. A test with high sensitivity means that a negative result rules out the target condition. Tests with high sensitivity are designed to identify everyone with a particular condition even if some people are identified who do not actually have the condition, i.e., false positives. Over-referral of these false positives is considered an acceptable outcome of screening and subsequent diagnostic testing eliminates them from receiving treatment.

Specificity

Specificity of a test is the proportion of individuals without the target condition who have a negative test result. In other words, specificity measures a test's ability to identify an individual without the disease as negative. Tests that are found to be highly specific indicate fewer false positive result and are able to help rule in the disorder of interest [14]. A test with high specificity means that a positive result rules in the patient as most likely having the target condition.

Positive and Negative Predictive Values

The accuracy of screening tests may also be reported in terms of predictive values. A positive predictive value is the probability that an individual with a positive, i.e., abnormal, test result actually has the target condition and represents the proportion of individuals who fail the screen and are identified as having the target condition based upon corroborating diagnostic testing. A negative predictive value is the probability that a person with a negative, i.e., normal, test result truly does not have the target condition and represents the proportion of individuals who pass the screen and are identified as not having the target condition based upon diagnostic testing.

False Positive and False Negative Rates

Accuracy of screening tests can also be described in terms of false positive and false negative rates. A false positive result occurs when the screen result is positive for an individual who does not have the condition being tested. The false positive rate is calculated as: $FP/(TP+FP)$. The ideal value for a false positive rate is 0. However, it is nearly impossible to achieve this when using a screening test in a large population.

A false negative result occurs when the screen reports a negative result for an individual who actually has the condition being screened. False negative rates are calculated as: $FN/(TN=FN)$.

- When evaluating the usefulness of a screening test the consequences of false positive and false negative rates need to be considered. Due to their inherent purpose screening tests have high sensitivities and low specificities. This allows for detection of most patients with aspiration risk while having the acceptable disadvantage of a high rate of false positives.

Likelihood Ratios

Another means of assessing accuracy of tests is the use of likelihood ratios. Likelihood ratios (LR) are defined as the likelihood that a given test result would be expected in an individual with the target disorder compared to the likelihood that the same result would be expected in an individual without the target disorder. One advantage likelihood ratios offer over sensitivity and specificity is that they are less likely to change due to the prevalence of a given disorder.

Likelihood ratios are expressed in terms of positive and negative likelihood ratios. A positive likelihood ratio indicates how the probability of a disease shifts when the finding is present. In other words, a positive likelihood ratio reflects the number of times it is more likely that a positive test comes from an individual with the disease rather than from an individual without the disease. A negative likelihood ratio indicates how the probability of disease shifts when it is absent. In other words, a negative likelihood ratio is equivalent to the number of times it is more likely that a negative test comes from an individual with the disease rather than from an individual without the disease.

Illustrative Example

To demonstrate how a 2×2 contingency table would be used to determine accuracy of a given screening test, let us suppose a hospital wants to implement a new screening procedure to determine if newly admitted patients are at risk for aspiration. The plan is to allow individuals who pass the screen to begin oral diets and oral medications without further instrumental evaluation. Patients who fail the screen will be referred for further testing. In this scenario, before the hospital can adopt the screen for use a determination must be made regarding the accuracy of the screen. To accomplish this, a pilot study is first performed with 100 individuals admitted with the diagnosis of suspected stroke. All participants in the pilot study complete both the screen followed immediately by an instrumental assessment of swallowing. The results are as follows:

		Aspiration on instrumental examination	
		Positive	Negative
Screening	Positive	a or True Positives (TP) $n = 50$	b or False Positives (FP) $n = 25$
	Negative	c or False Negatives (FN) $n = 2$	d or True Negatives (TN) $n = 23$

Sensitivity $= a/(a + c) = 50/(50 + 5) = 96.1\ \%$
Specificity $= d/(b + d) = 25/(25 + 23) = 52.1\ \%$
PPV $= a/(a + b) = 50/(50 + 25) = 66.7\ \%$
NPV $= d/(c + d) = 23/(2 + 23) = 92.0\ \%$
Positive Likelihood Ratio $=$ Sensitivity$/(1 -$ Specificity$)$
$= 0.961/1 - 0.521 = 2.006$
Negative Likelihood Ratio $= (1 -$ Sensitivity$)/$Specificity
$= (1 - 0.961)/.521 = 0.075$
False Positive Rate $=$ FP$/($TP $+$ FP$) = 25/(50 + 25) = 0.333$
False Negative Rate $=$ FN$/($TN $+$ FN$) = 2/(23 + 2) = 0.080$

In this scenario, the screening test results yield a high sensitivity (96.1 %) and a high negative predictive value (92 %), meaning that most individuals who passed the screen also did not aspirate on instrumental examination. This is a good result. Clinicians, therefore, can be confident that when patients pass the screen they are at very low aspiration risk and safe to begin oral alimentation. Specificity (52.1 %) and positive predictive value (66.7 %) for this screening test are considerably lower, indicating that many individuals who fail the screen (have a positive result) are not in actuality aspirating and will be referred for instrumental assessment unnecessarily. However, as previously discussed, over-referral is inherent in all screening instruments and is considered to be an acceptable limitation.

References

1. Streiner DL. Diagnosing tests: using and misusing diagnostic and screening tests. J Pers Assess. 2003;81:209–29.

2. Hafner G, Neuhuber A, Hirtenfelder S, Schmedler B, Eckel ME. Fiberoptic endoscopic evaluation of swallowing in intensive care unit patients. Eur Arch Otorhinolaryngol. 2008;265:441–6.
3. Heffner JE. Swallowing complications after endotracheal extubation. Chest. 2010;137:509–10.
4. de Larminat V, Montravers P, Dureuil B, Desmonts JM. Alteration in swallowing reflex extubation in intensive care unit patients. Crit Care Med. 1995;3:486–90.
5. Leder SB, Cohn SM, Moller BA. Fiberoptic endoscopic documentation of the high incidence of aspiration following extubation in critically ill trauma patients. Dysphagia. 1998;13:208–12.
6. Ajemian MS, Nirmul GB, Anderson MT, Zirlen DM, Kwasnik EM. Routine fiberoptic endoscopic evaluation of swallowing following prolonged intubation: implications for management. Arch Surg. 2001; 136:434–7.
7. Leder SB. Serial fiberoptic endoscopic swallowing examinations in the management of patients with dysphagia. Arch Phys Med Rehabil. 1998;79:1264–9.
8. Leder SB, Suiter DM, Lisitano HL. Answering orientation questions and following single step verbal commands: effect on aspiration status. Dysphagia. 2009;24:290–5.
9. Solh A, Okada M, Bhat A, Pietrantoni C. Swallowing disorders post orotracheal intubation in the elderly. Intensive Care Med. 2003; 29:1451–5.
10. Leder SB, Suiter DM. An epidemiologic study on aging and dysphagia in the acute care hospitalized population: 2000–2007. Gerontology. 2009;55:714–8.
11. Odderson IR, Keaton JC, McKenna BS. Swallow management in patients on an acute stroke pathway: quality is cost effective. Arch Phys Med Rehabil. 1995;76:1130–3.
12. Doggett DL, Tappe KA, Mitchell MD, Chapell R, Coates V, Turkelson CM. Prevention of pneumonia in elderly stroke patients by systematic diagnosis and treatment of dysphagia: an evidence-based comprehensive analysis of the literature. Dysphagia. 2001; 16:279–95.
13. Hinchey JA, Shephard T, Furie K, Smith D, Wang D, Tonn S. Formal dysphagia screening protocols prevent pneumonia. Stroke. 2005; 36:1972–6.
14. Rosenbek JC, McCullough GH, Wertz RT. Is the information about a test important? Applying the methods of evidence-based medicine to the clinical examination of swallowing. J Commun Disord. 2004;37:437–50.

Chapter 3
Criteria Necessary for a Successful and Reliable Swallow Screen

Objectives: To discuss why timely swallow screening with a reliable and validated swallow screen is important.

Methods: A targeted literature review regarding when and why to use a swallow screen are discussed.

Results: Supporting literature on timely use of a swallow screen and with patients requiring enteral tube feedings and tracheotomy tubes are discussed.

Conclusions: The Yale Swallow Protocol meets or exceeds all criteria required for a reliable and clinically useful swallow screen.

Keywords: Deglutition, Deglutition disorders, Swallow screening, Oral alimentation

Introduction

One of the keys to optimal patient care is use of a reliable and validated swallow screen. Criteria for a successful swallow screen are accuracy with a sensitivity of >95 % [1], use by a variety of trained health-care professionals, quick to perform, easy to interpret, cost effective, and, importantly, effective with virtually all patients regardless of diagnosis [2]. Use of such a screen saves both time and money as it relegates use of instrumental dysphagia testing

S.B. Leder and D.M. Suiter, *The Yale Swallow Protocol: An Evidence-Based Approach to Decision Making*, DOI 10.1007/978-3-319-05113-0_3, © Springer International Publishing Switzerland 2014

with FEES or VFSS only to patients who fail the swallow screen. The Yale Swallow Protocol (see Chap. 13) has been shown to fit all of these criteria.

The Yale Swallow Protocol has expanded upon prior research which used a 3-ounce water swallow in a small cohort ($n = 44$) of stroke patients [3]. The Yale Swallow Protocol, however, was validated using a much larger ($n = 3,000$) and more heterogeneous (14 distinct diagnostic categories) sample of hospitalized individuals [4]. It is comprised of a 3-ounce water swallow challenge [4], a brief cognitive screen [5], and an oral mechanism examination [6], with the latter two again using a large and heterogeneous sample of hospitalized individuals ($n = 4,102$).

The protocol requires drinking 3 ounces of water directly from a cup or via a straw without interruption. Criteria for failure are the inability to drink the entire volume, interrupted drinking, or coughing during drinking or immediately after completion of drinking. The cognitive screen requires answers to three orientation questions: (1) What is your name? (2) Where are you right now? (3) What year is it? And following three single-step verbal commands: (1) Open your mouth, (2) Stick out your tongue, and (3) Smile [5]. The oral mechanism examination includes visual assessment of adequate labial closure, lingual range of motion, and facial symmetry (smile/pucker) [6].

Heffner [7] suggested using the Yale Swallow Protocol because of its robust operating characteristics. To wit, aspiration risk was determined with 96.5 % sensitivity [4], 97.9 % negative predictive value [4], and a <2 % false negative rate [8]. Importantly, when the protocol was passed a 100 % success rate with subsequent oral alimentation was observed [9–11]. Therefore, when combined with the clinical judgment of an experienced clinician, both aspiration risk and oral diet recommendations can be confidently determined in virtually all patients who are deemed potential candidates for oral intake [11]. Recommendations for continued nil-per-os status, repeat protocol administration, referral for instrumental dysphagia testing, or initiation of foods, fluids, and medications can be made safely and in a timely manner for optimal patient care.

There is no harm, and a distinct benefit, to timely screening. Many times a patient will pass who, at first blush, did not appear capable, resulting in timely and safe resumption of oral alimentation. Repeat screening at 24-h intervals can be done, also without harm, prior to recommending instrumental testing. Since many hospitalized patients often demonstrate rapid improvement in their medical condition, including swallowing function [12], whenever the protocol is passed diet recommendations can be confidently made without the need for instrumental dysphagia testing.

If a second or even a third swallow protocol failure occurs, however, instrumental testing is required to determine when to resume safe oral alimentation and with what type of food consistencies. FEES is advantageous to use because in-the-room bedside testing precludes transport to diagnostic radiology resulting in minimal disruption to patient care. VFSS should be performed if trans-nasal endoscopy is contraindicated or there is a question of esophageal dysphagia. FEES testing was shown to be highly beneficial as 71 % of patients who failed the protocol were nonetheless able to eat a modified consistency oral diet safely, e.g., nectar-like thickened liquid and puree consistency foods and/or compensatory strategies of limiting to single small (5–10 cc) bolus volumes [4].

What About Non-swallowing Stimuli?

Can non-swallowing variables be used to determine aspiration risk? A systematic literature review from 1950 to 2009 of 1,489 manuscripts did not find a single reliable non-swallowing variable that was associated with an increased swallowing or aspiration risk in critically ill patients [13]. Specifically, the variables of age, gender, diagnosis, duration of intubation, and timing of post-extubation swallowing assessments were all *unreliable* predictors of aspiration risk. Since determination of an a priori aspiration risk based upon non-swallowing indicators is not supported in an evidence-based fashion, it is of upmost importance to assess for aspiration risk with a swallowing task. The Yale Swallow Protocol was designed precisely for this reason.

Can Testing Be Done with Nasogastric and Orogastric Feeding Tubes in Place?

Can enteral tube feedings continue during swallowing testing? Nasogastric tubes, either small- or large-bore [14, 15], and large-bore orogastric tubes [16], all commonly used in hospitalized patients, were previously anecdotally believed to impact on swallowing success. Subsequent research has shown that there is no causal effect on dysphagia or aspiration status from nasogastric or orogastric tube use [14–16]. Despite the fact that both nasogastric and orogastric tubes traverse the same pathway as a food bolus, the presence or absence of either tube and either size did not affect incidence of aspiration or aspiration dependent upon food consistency, i.e., liquid or puree [14, 15]. Importantly, it is neither necessary to remove a nasogastric or orogastric tube to evaluate aspiration status nor is it contraindicated to leave either tube in place to supplement oral alimentation until prandial nutrition is adequate [14–16].

What About Tracheotomy Tubes?

Many hospitalized patients require a tracheotomy tube for airway maintenance. Previously, increased aspiration risk was erroneously attributed to a tracheotomy and placement of a tracheotomy tube. More recent research on swallowing and aspiration status pre- and post-tracheotomy in the same individual clearly demonstrated no causal relationship between tracheotomy and placement of a tracheotomy tube and aspiration status. Specifically, the presence or absence of a tracheotomy tube has been shown to be irrelevant to swallowing success or failure [17, 18]. Rather, it is the underlying medical condition that necessitated a tracheotomy in the first place that is the cause of the observed dysphagia and aspiration.

Caveat Regarding the Yale Swallow Protocol and Tracheotomy Tube Use

An important caveat, however, is that the Yale Swallow Protocol, which includes a 3-ounce water swallow challenge, should not be used for screening patients who require a tracheotomy tube. Silent aspiration occurs more frequently due to laryngeal desensitization from airflow bypassing the upper airway and chronic aspiration of secretions [19, 20]. Although neither a tracheotomy nor a tracheotomy tube is causal for aspiration [17, 18] if aspiration occurs it is often silent leading to potentially higher false negative rates. Therefore, it is recommended that instrumental testing with either FEES or VFSS be done with patients who require a tracheotomy tube. All other medical and surgical patients, however, are candidates for the Yale Swallow Protocol.

Importance of Clinical Judgment

The combined clinical judgment and experience of the hospitalist, intensivist, and speech-language pathologist are essential in the care of the hospitalized individual with suspected aspiration risk. In addition to appropriate referral for and administration of the Yale Swallow Protocol, further patient-specific factors need to be taken into account in order for screening to be as accurate as possible and recommendations for an oral diet safe and successful. Optimal administration and interpretation of the Yale Swallow Protocol requires knowledge of pre-morbid feeding status and ability; current cognitive abilities, cooperativeness, and level of consciousness; gross oral motor skills; respiratory issues; and any positioning and posture limitations. When an experienced clinician assesses the patient in such a holistic manner the already excellent operating characteristics of the Yale Swallow Protocol, i.e., sensitivity 96.5 %, negative predictive value 97.9 %, and <2 % false negative rate, may improve and thereby strengthen protocol results. However, failure to account for these important factors may lead to an inappropriately high failure rate and unnecessary instrumental dysphagia testing.

References

1. Leder SB, Espinosa JF. Aspiration risk after acute stroke: comparison of clinical examination and fiberoptic endoscopic evaluation of swallowing. Dysphagia. 2002;17:214–8.
2. Cochrane AL, Holland WW. Validation of screening procedures. British Med Bull. 1971;27:3–8.

3. DePippo KL, Holas MA, Reding MJ. Validation of the 3-oz water swallow test for aspiration following stroke. Arch Neurol. 1992;49:1259–61.

4. Suiter DB, Leder SB. Clinical utility of the 3 ounce water swallow test. Dysphagia. 2008;23:244–50.

5. Leder SB, Suiter DM, Warner HL. Answering orientation questions and following single step verbal commands: effect on aspiration status. Dysphagia. 2009;24:290–5.

6. Leder SB, Suiter DM, Murray J, Rademaker AW. Can an oral mechanism examination contribute to the assessment of odds of aspiration? Dysphagia. 2013;28:370–4.

7. Heffner JE. Swallowing complications after endotracheal extubation. Chest. 2010;137:509–10.

8. Leder SB, Suiter DM, Green BG. Silent aspiration risk is volume dependent. Dysphagia. 2011;26:304–9.

9. Leder SB, Suiter DM, Warner HL, Kaplan LJ. Initiating safe oral feeding in critically ill intensive care and step-down unit patients based on passing a 3-ounce (90 milliliters) water swallow challenge. J Trauma. 2011;70:1203–7.

10. Leder SB, Suiter DM, Warner HL, Acton LM, Swainson BA. Success of recommending oral diets in acute stroke patients based on a 90-cc water swallow challenge protocol. Top Stroke Rehabil. 2012;19:40–4.

11. Leder SB, Suiter DM, Warner HL, Acton LM, Siegel MD. Safe initiation of oral diets in hospitalized patients based on passing a 3-ounce (90 cc) water swallow challenge protocol. Q J Med. 2012;105:257–63.

12. Leder SB. Serial fiberoptic endoscopic swallowing evaluations in the management of patients with dysphagia. Arch Phys Med Rehabil. 1998; 79:1264–9.

13. Skoretz SA, Flowers HL, Martino R. The incidence of dysphagia following endotracheal intubation. Chest. 2010;137:665–73.

14. Leder SB, Suiter DM. Effect of nasogastric tubes on incidence of aspiration. Arch Phys Med Rehabil. 2008;89:648–51.

15. Fattal M, Suiter DM, Warner HL, Leder SB. Effect of presence/absence of a nasogastric tube in the same person on incidence of aspiration. Otolaryngol Head Neck Surg. 2011;145:796–800.

16. Leder SB, Lazarus CL, Suiter DM, Acton LM. Effect of orogastric tubes on aspiration status and recommendations for oral feeding. Otolaryngol Head Neck Surg. 2011;144:372–5.

17. Leder SB, Ross DA. Investigation of the causal relationship between tracheotomy and aspiration in the acute care setting. Laryngoscope. 2000; 110:641–4.

18. Leder SB, Ross DA. Confirmation of no causal relationship between tracheotomy and aspiration status: a direct replication study. Dysphagia. 2010;25:35–9.

19. Link DT, Willging JP, Miller CK. Pediatric laryngopharyngeal sensory testing during flexible endoscopic evaluation of swallowing: feasible and correlative. Ann Otol Rhinol Laryngol. 2000;109:899–905.

20. Donzelli J, Brady S, Wesling M. Predictive value of accumulated oropharyngeal secretions for aspiration during video nasal endoscopic evaluation of swallowing. Ann Otol Rhinol Laryngol. 2003;112:469–75.

Chapter 4
Development of a Programmatic Line of Research for Swallow Screening for Aspiration Risk: The First Step

Suiter DM, Leder SB. Clinical utility of the 3 ounce water swallow test. Dysphagia 2008;23:244–50. (Used and modified with kind permission from Springer Science + Business Media.)

A number of studies have used 3 ounces of water to screen for aspiration risk [1–4]. However, the sample sizes were both small and homogeneous, the methodologies different, and, importantly, no corroborating evidence was presented linking a successful 3-ounce water swallow challenge with swallowing success of different consistencies such as puree and solid food. There would be limited benefit to passing any screen if diet recommendations could not be implemented without the need for further dysphagia testing. In other words, why screen at all if an instrumental test is still required before starting oral alimentation. In order for the 3-ounce challenge to be the foundation of the Yale Swallow Protocol both its sensitivity and negative predictive value must be >95 % [5].

Objectives: The 3-ounce water swallow challenge is frequently used when screening individuals for aspiration risk. Prior research concerning its clinical usefulness, however, is confounded by inadequate statistical power due to small and homogeneous sample sizes and varying methodologies. Importantly, research has been limited to a select patient population, i.e., stroke, thereby limiting its widespread generalizability and applicability. Our purpose was to investigate the clinical utility of the 3-ounce water swallow challenge to determine aspiration risk status as well as oral feeding recommendations in a large and heterogeneous hospitalized patient population.

Methods: In order to do this, FEES was performed in conjunction with the 3-ounce challenge with 3,000 participants presenting from 14 different diagnostic categories. A total of 1,151 (38.4 %) participants passed and 1,849 (61.6 %) failed the 3-ounce water swallow challenge.

Results: Sensitivity of the 3-ounce water swallow challenge for predicting aspiration status during FEES was 96.5 % with a negative predictive value of 97.9 %. Sensitivity for identifying individuals who were deemed safe for oral intake based on FEES results was 96.4 % with a negative predictive value of 98.3 %. Passing the 3-ounce water swallow test appears to be a good predictor of ability to tolerate thin liquids *and* a good predictor of ability to eat and drink. However, when used as an isolated variable in the determination of aspiration risk, failure on the 3-ounce challenge often does not indicate inability to tolerate thin liquids due to a low specificity of 48.7 %. Similar to all other swallow screens isolated use of the 3-ounce water swallow challenge to make decisions regarding safety of liquid intake results in over-referral. Specifically, 71 % of participants who failed the challenge were nevertheless deemed safe for some type of oral diet or feeding modification based on FEES.

Conclusions: The important finding is that since FEES was performed in conjunction with the challenge if the 3-ounce water swallow challenge is passed, diet recommendations can be made without further instrumental dysphagia testing.

Keywords: Deglutition, Deglutition disorders, Aspiration risk, Dysphagia screening, Oral alimentation

Introduction

Accurate identification of individuals with potential aspiration risk is critically important because of the high incidence of pneumonia associated with unrecognized prandial aspiration [6]. As discussed in Chap. 2, any clinically useful screening test for aspiration risk should provide both high sensitivity and high negative predictive value [7]. The goal is accurate identification of individuals who aspirate and require further testing while ruling out non-aspirators who do not require intervention. To be useful in clinical practice a screening test for determination of aspiration risk should have three goals:

1. To determine the likelihood that aspiration risk is present.
2. To determine the need for an objective swallow evaluation.
3. To determine when it is safe to recommend resumption of oral alimentation.

However, the optimal means of screening individuals with potential aspiration risk is fraught with poor methodology, inadequate sample sizes, and use of nonevidence-based stimuli [1–4, 8–20].

The task of drinking 3 ounces of water was one of the first published methods used for screening individuals for aspiration risk [2]. The task requires drinking 3 ounces of water completely, without interruption, and without coughing or choking. Criteria for referral for further assessment of swallowing include inability to complete the task, interrupted drinking, or coughing or choking. Although the contribution of the 3-ounce water swallow challenge to the detection of aspiration risk during clinical (bedside) swallowing screening has been reported [2, 3, 12, 14, 17], the evidence is unconvincing because of inadequate statistical power due to small sample sizes, homogeneity of population samples, and varying methodologies.

The clinical utility of the 3-ounce water swallow challenge has focused primarily on adult individuals following a stroke. Studies have reported variable sensitivity and specificity results [2, 3, 12, 14, 17], ranging from a sensitivity as high as 86 % but with specificity as low as 50 % [17]. The clinical usefulness of the 3-ounce challenge in larger and more heterogeneous patient populations is vitally important for implementation to widespread patient care.

Three Research Questions

Therefore, we examined the clinical usefulness of the 3-ounce water swallow challenge for determining both aspiration risk status and oral feeding recommendations in a much larger and

TABLE 4.1.   Participant demographic information.

Gender[a]	Males	Females
	$N=1,669$ (55.6 %)	$N=1,324$ (44.3 %)
Age[b]	$\bar{X}=66.8$ year	$\bar{X}=70.14$ year
	(Range=2.2–105.0 year)	(Range=3.0–105.0 year)

With kind permission from Springer Science + Business Media: Suiter DM, Leder SB. Clinical utility of the 3 ounce water swallow test. Dysphagia 2008;23:244–250
[a]Data are missing for 7 (.2 %) of participants
[b]Data are missing for 18 (.6 %) of participants

more heterogeneous population sample. Three research questions were posed:

1. Does the 3-ounce water swallow challenge identify individuals who aspirate thin liquids?
2. Does a failed 3-ounce water swallow challenge identify individuals who are also unsafe for oral alimentation based on results of an instrumental swallow assessment?
3. If the 3-ounce water swallow challenge is passed, can specific oral diet recommendations be made without further instrumental assessment?

All FEES performed from December, 1999 to September, 2006 were included. Data from a total of 3,000 inpatients from a large, urban, tertiary care, teaching hospital were analyzed. Table 4.1 shows participant demographics and Fig. 4.1 shows number of participants by age.

The standard FEES protocol was followed with slight modifications [21, 22]. Briefly, each naris was examined visually and the scope passed through the most patent naris without administration of a topical anesthetic or vasoconstrictor to the nasal mucosa, thereby eliminating any potential adverse anesthetic reaction and assuring the endoscopist of a safe physiologic examination [23]. The base of tongue, pharynx, and larynx were viewed and swallowing was evaluated directly with six food boluses of approximately 5 mL volume each.

The first food challenge consisted of three boluses of puree consistency (yellow pudding) followed by three liquid boluses

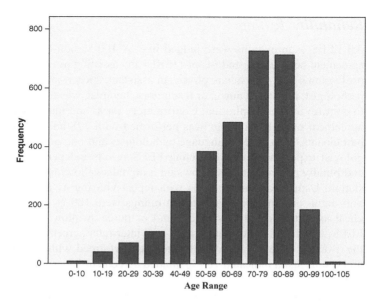

FIG. 4.1. Participant ages by decade. (With kind permission from Springer Science + Business Media: Suiter DM, Leder SB. Clinical utility of the 3 ounce water swallow test. Dysphagia 2008;23:244–250).

(white milk), as these colors have excellent contrast with pharyngeal and laryngeal mucosa [24]. Aspiration was defined as entry of material into the airway below the level of the true vocal folds [25] and silent aspiration occurred when there were no external behavioral signs such as coughing or choking [26]. A safe swallow was defined as no aspiration during FEES.

Immediately following completion of FEES, the same investigator (SBL) administered the 3-ounce water swallow challenge. Each participant was given 3 ounces of water and asked to drink without interruption, and results were recorded. Criteria for challenge failure included inability to drink the entire amount, interrupted drinking, or coughing during or immediately after completion.

Reliability Testing

All FEES examinations were judged live. A 100 % non-blinded agreement between the endoscopist (SBL) and assisting health-care professional, e.g., physician, physician assistant, speech-language pathologist, registered nurse, or respiratory therapist, was required to confirm tracheal aspiration. Confirmatory intra- and inter-rater agreement of FEES findings was performed with 128 additional participants. Two speech-language pathologists and one otolaryngologist experienced in interpreting FEES results independently and blindly reviewed the swallows on a digital swallowing workstation. Using real-time analysis with repeat viewing as needed, both intra- and inter-rater agreement ratings were 100 % for tracheal aspiration on at least one liquid or puree swallow during FEES. Additional confirmatory intra- and inter-rater agreement for the 3-ounce water swallow challenge was performed with VFSS and results again indicated 100 % blinded agreement for aspiration status [27].

FEES results served as the outcome variable and were the criterion standard to which results of the 3-ounce water swallow challenge were compared. A 2×2 contingency table was used to evaluate results of the challenge. If aspiration was present on FEES when a participant failed the water swallow test, a *true positive* rating resulted. If aspiration was not present on FEES when a participant passed the water swallow test, a *true negative* rating resulted. If aspiration was not present on FEES but the participant failed the water swallow test, a *false positive* rating resulted. If aspiration was present on FEES but the participant passed the water swallow test, a *false negative* rating resulted.

The diagnostic value of a test can be expressed by means of its sensitivity and specificity. Sensitivity was computed by dividing the number of participants with a true positive result on the water swallow test by the total number of participants who aspirated on FEES. Specificity was computed by dividing the number of participants with a true negative result on the water swallow test by the total number of participants who did not aspirate on FEES. Positive predictive value was computed by dividing the number of participants with a true positive result on the water swallow test by the total number of participants who failed the water swallow test. Negative predictive value was computed by dividing the number of participants with a true negative result on the water swallow test by the number of participants who passed the water swallow test. Positive likelihood ratio was computed by dividing sensitivity by 1 minus the specificity. Negative likelihood ratio was computed by dividing 1 minus sensitivity by specificity. (See Chap. 2 for an in-depth explanation of statistical terms used with screening tests.)

Answers to the Three Research Questions

3-Ounce Water Swallow Challenge and Liquid Aspiration Based on FEES Results

The answer to our first research question, "Does the 3-ounce water swallow challenge identify individuals who aspirate thin liquids?" is provided in Table 4.2. A total of 1,151 of 3,000 participants (38.4 %) passed the 3-ounce water swallow challenge.

TABLE 4.2. 2×2 Contingency table demonstrating sensitivity, specificity, positive predictive value, negative predictive value, positive likelihood ratio, and negative likelihood ratio of the 3-ounce water swallow test for detecting aspiration.

		Aspiration on FEES	
		Positive	Negative
3-Ounce water test	Positive	664	1,185
		a = True Positive	b = False Positive
	Negative	24	1,127
		c = False Negative	d = True Negative

With kind permission from Springer Science + Business Media: Suiter DM, Leder SB. Clinical utility of the 3 ounce water swallow test. Dysphagia 2008;23:244–250

Sensitivity = $a/(a+c) = 664/(664+24) = 96.5$ % (95 % CI = 94.9–97.6)

Specificity = $d/(b+d) = 1127/(1185+1127) = 48.7$ % (95 % CI = 48.3–49.1)

Positive Predictive Value = $a/(a+b) = 664/(664+1185) = 35.9$ % (95 % CI = 35.3–36.3)

Negative Predictive Value = $d/(c+d) = 1127/(24+1127) = 97.9$ % (95 % CI = 97.0–98.6)

Positive Likelihood Ratio = sensitivity/(1 − specificity) = 0.965/(1−0.487) = 1.883 (95 % CI = 1.835–1.917)

Negative Likelihood Ratio = 1 − sensitivity/specificity = (1 − 0.965)/0.487 = 0.072 (95 % CI = 0.048–0.105)

A total of 1,849 of 3,000 (61.6 %) individuals failed the 3-ounce water swallow challenge. Despite failure on the 3-ounce water swallow challenge, 1,029 of 1,849 (55.7 %) participants were able to tolerate thin liquids based on FEES results. Additionally, 254 of 1,849 (13.7 %) individuals who failed the water challenge were deemed safe for modified liquid intake, i.e., thickened liquids. Finally, 565 of 1,849 (30.6 %) individuals who failed the water swallow challenge were also deemed to be unsafe for liquid intake based on FEES results.

To determine if the 3-ounce water swallow challenge was a reliable predictor of aspiration dependent upon medical diagnosis, sensitivity, specificity, positive predictive value, and negative predictive value were calculated for individuals in 14 diagnostic categories. Results of these analyses are presented in Table 4.3. Sensitivity ranged from 90.9 % for individuals who were post-esophageal surgery to 100.0 % for individuals who were post head and neck surgery, neurosurgery, brainstem stroke, Parkinson's disease, and dementia. Specificity ranged from 25.4 % for individuals with dementia to 67.3 % for those who were post-esophageal surgery. Positive predictive value ranged from 22.1 % for individuals with dementia to 62.9 % for individuals who were post head and neck surgery. Negative predictive values were con- siderably higher, ranging from 94.9 % for individuals who were post cardiothoracic surgery to 100.0 % for individuals in 5 diag- nostic categories including those who were status post neurosur- gery and those with brainstem stroke.

3-Ounce Water Swallow Test and Diet Recommendations Based on FEES Results

The answer to our second research question, "Does a failed 3-ounce water swallow challenge identify individuals who are also unsafe for oral alimentation based on results of an instrumen- tal swallow assessment?" is provided in Table 4.4. To determine if the 3-ounce water swallow challenge was a reliable predictor of oral intake status dependent upon medical diagnosis, sensitivity, specificity, positive predictive value, and negative predictive

TABLE 4.3. Water test and liquid aspiration by diagnostic category with 95 % confidence intervals.

	SENS	SPEC	PPV	NPV	+LR	−LR
Cardiothoracic surgery (N=180)	95.5 (88.5–98.4)	49.1 (45.1–50.8)	52.1 (48.3–53.7)	94.9 (87.2–98.2)	1.88 (1.61–2.20)	0.09 (0.03–0.25)
Esophageal surgery (N=63)	90.9 (65.3–98.4)	67.3 (61.9–68.9)	37.0 (26.6–40.1)	97.2 (89.4–99.5)	2.78 (1.71–3.16)	0.14 (0.02–0.56)
Head and Neck surgery (N=111)	100.0 (94.7–100.0)	40.0 (34.6–40.0)	62.9 (59.6–62.9)	1.00 (86.5–1.00)	1.67 (1.45–1.67)	0.00 (0.00–0.15)
Neurosurgery (N=232)	100.0 (93.6–100.0)	42.2 (40.4–42.2)	33.3 (31.2–33.3)	100.0 (95.6–100.0)	1.73 (1.57–1.73)	0.00 (0.00–0.16)
Medical (N=492)	95.0 (89.9–97.7)	51.1 (49.4–51.9)	38.5 (36.4–39.6)	96.9 (93.8–98.6)	1.94 (1.78–2.03)	0.10 (0.05–0.20)
Pulmonary (N=451)	96.1 (91.5–98.3)	54.0 (52.2–54.9)	45.0 (42.5–46.1)	97.2 (94.0–98.8)	2.09 (1.91–2.18)	0.07 (0.03–0.16)
Cancer (N=125)	93.8 (81.5–98.2)	53.8 (49.6–55.3)	41.1 (35.7–43.1)	96.2 (88.6–98.9)	2.03 (1.62–2.20)	0.12 (0.03–0.37)
Other (N=391)	97.5 (91.7–99.3)	58.2 (56.7–58.7)	37.5 (35.3–38.2)	98.9 (96.4–99.7)	2.33 (2.12–2.40)	0.04 (0.01–0.15)
Left stroke (N=227)	97.8 (89.3–99.6)	45.3 (43.1–45.8)	31.3 (28.5–31.8)	98.8 (94.1–99.8)	1.79 (1.57–1.84)	0.05 (0.01–0.25)
Right stroke (N=203)	92.7 (81.7–97.4)	40.7 (38.0–41.9)	28.4 (25.0–29.8)	95.7 (89.1–98.5)	1.56 (1.32–1.68)	0.18 (0.06–0.48)
Brainstem stroke (N=38)	100.0 (68.5–100.0)	54.8 (47.7–54.8)	33.3 (22.8–33.3)	100.0 (87.0–100.0)	2.21 (1.31–2.21)	0.00 (0.00–0.67)
Parkinson's disease (N=18)	100.0 (69.2–100.0)	58.3 (42.9–58.3)	54.5 (37.7–54.5)	100.0 (73.6–100.0)	2.40 (1.21–2.40)	0.00 (0.00–0.72)
Dementia (N=86)	100.0 (82.2–100.0)	25.4 (21.6–25.4)	22.1 (1.81–22.1)	100.0 (85.2–100.0)	1.34 (1.05–1.34)	0.00 (0.00–0.82)
Other Neuro. (N=364)	97.1 (92.1–99.0)	43.1 (37.3–45.4)	45.2 (42.9–46.1)	97.9 (94.4–99.3)	2.12 (1.93–2.20)	0.05 (0.02–0.15)

With kind permission from Springer Science+Business Media: Suiter DM, Leder SB. Clinical utility of the 3 ounce water swallow test. Dysphagia 2008;23:244-250

SENS Sensitivity, *SPEC* Specificity, *PPV* Positive Predictive Value, *NPV* Negative Predictive Value, *+LR* Positive Likelihood Ratio, *−LR* Negative Likelihood Ratio

TABLE 4.4. 2×2 contingency table demonstrating sensitivity, specificity, positive predictive value, negative predictive value, positive likelihood ratio, and negative likelihood ratio of the 3-ounce water swallow test for ability to tolerate oral diet.

		Aspiration on FEES	
		Positive	Negative
3-Ounce water test	Positive	543	1,304
		a = True Positive	b = False Positive
	Negative	20	1,131
		c = False Negative	d = True Negative

With kind permission from Springer Science + Business Media: Suiter DM, Leder SB. Clinical utility of the 3 ounce water swallow test. Dysphagia 2008;23:244–250

Sensitivity = a/(a + c) = 543/(543 + 20) = 96.4 % (95 % CI = 94.6–97.7)

Specificity = d/(b + d) = 1131/(1304 + 1131) = 46.4 % (95 % CI = 46.0–46.7)

Positive Predictive Value = a/(a + b) = 543/(543 + 1304) = 29.4 % (95 % CI = 28.8–29.8)

Negative Predictive Value = d/(c + d) = 1131/(20 + 1131) = 98.3 % (95 % CI = 97.4–98.9)

Positive Likelihood Ratio = sensitivity/(1 − specificity) = .964/(1–0.464) = 1.801 (95 % CI = 1.753–1.834)

Negative Likelihood Ratio = 1 − sensitivity/specificity = (1–0.964)/0.464 = 0.076 (95 % CI = 0.050–0.117)

value were calculated for individuals in 14 diagnostic categories. Results are presented in Table 4.5, and the same pattern as in Table 4.3 was observed.

To answer to our third research question, "If the 3-ounce water swallow challenge is passed, can specific diet recommendations be made without further swallow assessment?," a cross tabulation examining diet recommendation and water test results was performed. *It is important to note that all diet recommendations were based on FEES results.* Of the 1,151 participants who passed the 3-ounce water swallow challenge, 648 of 1,151 (56 %) were cleared for a regular diet; 147 of 1,151 (13 %) were cleared for a soft diet; 45 of 1,151 (4 %) were cleared for a chopped diet; 289 of 1,151 (25 %) were cleared for a puree diet; and 3 of 1,151 (0.3 %) were cleared for a liquid diet. Twenty of 1,151 (1.5 %), although passing the water swallow challenge, were made nil by mouth based on FEES results, i.e., false negatives. Despite failure on the 3-ounce water swallow challenge, 1,304 of 1,849 participants (70.5 %) were nonetheless able to tolerate either a modified consistency oral diet,

TABLE 4.5. Water test and diet recommendations by diagnostic category with 95 % confidence intervals.

	SENS	SPEC	PPV	NPV	+LR	−LR
Cardiothoracic Surgery (N=178)	96.0 (87.6–98.9)	44.5 (41.2–45.7)	40.3 (36.8–41.5)	96.6 (89.5–99.1)	1.73 (1.49–1.82)	0.09 (0.02–0.30)
Esophageal Surgery (N=62)	87.5 (55.4–97.7)	64.8 (60.1–66.3)	26.9 (17.1–30.1)	97.2 (90.1–99.5)	2.49 (1.39–2.90)	0.19 (0.03–0.74)
Head and Neck Surgery (N=111)	100.0 (93.7–100.0)	34.4 (29.7–34.4)	52.8 (49.5–52.8)	1.00 (86.5–1.00)	1.52 (1.33–1.52)	0.00 (0.00–0.21)
Neurosurgery (N=232)	100.0 (92.8–100.0)	40.9 (39.1–40.9)	29.5 (23.0–29.5)	100.0 (95.6–100.0)	1.69 (1.52–1.69)	0.00 (0.00–0.19)
Medical (N=491)	94.5 (88.2–97.6)	47.8 (46.3–48.5)	29.2 (27.2–30.1)	97.4 (94.5–98.9)	1.81 (1.64–1.89)	0.12 (0.05–0.26)
Pulmonary (N=450)	93.9 (87.0–97.3)	47.6 (46.0–48.3)	28.5 (26.4–29.6)	97.2 (94.1–98.8)	1.79 (1.61–1.88)	0.13 (0.06–0.28)
Cancer (N=125)	93.5 (80.9–98.2)	53.2 (49.0–54.7)	39.7 (34.4–41.7)	96.2 (88.6–98.9)	2.00 (1.59–2.17)	0.12 (0.03–0.39)
Other (N=391)	96.2 (87.4–99.0)	53.4 (52.1–53.8)	24.0 (21.9–24.7)	98.9 (96.4–99.7)	2.06 (1.82–2.14)	0.07 (0.02–0.24)
Left Stroke (N=229)	96.3 (82.5–99.3)	41.1 (39.2–41.5)	17.9 (15.4–18.5)	98.8 (94.4–99.8)	1.64 (1.36–1.70)	0.09 (0.02–0.45)
Right Stroke (N=202)	95.8 (80.7–99.3)	38.2 (36.2–38.7)	17.3 (14.6–17.9)	98.6 (93.3–99.7)	1.55 (1.27–1.62)	0.11 (0.02–0.53)
Brainstem Stroke (N=39)	100.0 (71.6–100.0)	58.1 (50.7–58.1)	38.1 (27.3–38.1)	100.0 (87.4–100.0)	2.39 (1.45–2.39)	0.00 (0.00–0.56)
Parkinson's Disease (N=18)	100.0 (57.5–100.0)	50.0 (37.8–50.0)	36.4 (20.9–36.4)	100.0 (75.7–100.0)	2.00 (0.94–2.00)	0.00 (0.00–1.12)
Dementia (N=87)	100.0 (81.1–100.0)	24.7 (21.0–24.7)	20.3 (16.5–20.3)	100.0 (85.3–100.0)	1.33 (1.03–1.33)	0.00 (0.00–0.90)
Other Neuro. (N=364)	98.7 (93.1–99.8)	49.8 (48.4–50.1)	33.8 (31.9–34.2)	99.3 (96.4–99.9)	1.97 (1.80–2.00)	0.03 (0.00–0.14)

With kind permission from Springer Science + Business Media: Suiter DM, Leder SB. Clinical utility of the 3 ounce water swallow test. Dysphagia 2008;23:244–250
SENS Sensitivity, *SPEC* Specificity, *PPV* Positive Predictive Value, *NPV* Negative Predictive Value, *+LR* Positive Likelihood Ratio, *−LR* Negative Likelihood Ratio

e.g., nectar-like thickened liquids, or swallow strategies, e.g., single small <5 cc bolus volumes, based on FEES results. The remaining 545 of 3,000 participants (18 %) were made nil per os.

Synthesizing and Discussing the Results

These results support the purpose of our study, i.e., to determine the clinical utility of the 3-ounce water swallow challenge for determining both aspiration risk status and ability to recommend an oral diet in a large and heterogeneous population sample. The 3-ounce challenge was sensitive for determining aspiration risk of thin liquids as confirmed by instrumental assessment since 96.6 % of participants who aspirated on FEES also failed the water swallow challenge. In addition, the 3-ounce water swallow challenge had a high negative predictive value of 97.9 % which indicated that most individuals who passed the water swallow challenge, i.e., had a negative response, also did not aspirate during instrumental examination. In the vast majority of cases, therefore, passing the 3-ounce water swallow challenge is a good predictor of determining both a patient's aspiration risk and a patient's ability to safely tolerate not only thin liquids but also other food consistencies.

The clinical utility of the 3-ounce water swallow challenge for determining whether an individual could safely tolerate oral intake was supported. Results were similar to those for liquid aspiration risk. The 3-ounce water swallow challenge was a sensitive test with a high negative predictive rate for determining an individual's ability to safely tolerate oral intake. However, because nearly 71 % of participants who failed the isolated water swallow challenge were nonetheless deemed safe for some form of oral intake based on results of FEES, failure on the isolated 3-ounce water swallow challenge did not accurately reflect true oral feeding status.

Prior to the present study, there were no data to support recommendations for an oral diet based on a successful 3-ounce water swallow challenge. In actuality, passing the 3-ounce water swallow challenge only indicated that thin liquids were tolerated, and an instrumental dysphagia evaluation was needed anyway to determine diet recommendations and feeding safety for puree or solid food consistencies [6]. Therefore, for the first time with objective (FEES) data, we have shown that if the challenge was passed patients can be recommended an oral diet safely and without further instrumental dysphagia testing. Specifically, a puree diet is usually recommended for edentulous patients and a soft or regular consistency diet is usually recommended for dentate patients.

We must stress that clinical judgment and experience, in conjunction with objective information, are essential factors in the care of the individual with suspected aspiration risk. Although the vast majority of patients (i.e., 1,134 of 1,151 [98.5 %]) who passed the 3-ounce water swallow challenge were recommended for and successful with oral alimentation, additional patient-specific factors must be taken into consideration in order for an oral diet to be safe and successful. For example, the clinician must be aware that patients with dementia need to be evaluated regarding following directions and self-feeding skills, patients with stroke require assessment for neglect, limb apraxia, and nondominant upper extremity use, patients with traumatic brain injury need to be monitored regarding impulsivity and task attentiveness, and patients who are deconditioned and easily fatigued require diet modifications and assistance with eating. All patients with swallowing difficulties benefit from encouragement and monitoring as work toward the goal of normal eating progresses. The dysphagia specialist, therefore, must synthesize objective, subjective, and behavioral data on an individual basis to promote safe and successful eating.

Conclusions

In conclusion, results of this study have expanded the clinical usefulness of the 3-ounce water swallow challenge. Importantly, when the challenge is passed, not only thin liquids but also other food consistencies can be recommended confidently and without further instrumental dysphagia assessment. That is, following a successful 3-ounce water swallow challenge, and taking into consideration any patient-specific factors that may impact on resumption of safe oral intake, recommendations for specific diet consistencies can be made, e.g., puree, chopped, soft-solid, or regular diet.

References

1. DePippo KL, Holas MA, Reding MJ. The burke dysphagia screening test: validation of its use in patients with stroke. Arch Phys Med Rehabil. 1994;75:1284–6.
2. DePippo KL, Holas MA, Reding MJ. Validation of the 3-oz water swallow test for aspiration following stroke. Arch Neurol. 1992;49:1259–61.
3. Garon BR, Engle M, Ormiston C. Reliability of the 3-oz water swallow test utilizing cough reflex as sole indicator of aspiration. Neurorehabil Neural Repair. 1995;9:139–43.
4. McCullough GH, Wertz RT, Rosenbek JC. Sensitivity and specificity of clinical/bedside examination signs for detecting aspiration in adults subsequent to stroke. J Commun Disord. 2001;34:55–72.
5. Leder SB, Espinosa JF. Aspiration risk after acute stroke: comparison of clinical examination and fiberoptic endoscopic evaluation of swallowing. Dysphagia. 2002;17:214–8.
6. Langmore SE, Terpenning MS, Schork A, Chen Y, Murray JT, Lopatin D, Loesche WJ. Predictors of aspiration pneumonia: how important is dysphagia? Dysphagia. 1998;13:69–81.
7. Fletcher RH, Fletcher SW, Wagner EH. Clinical epidemiology: the essentials. Baltimore: Williams & Wilkins; 1988.
8. Chong MS, Lieu PK, Sitoh YY, Meng YY, Leow LP. Bedside clinical methods useful as screening test for aspiration in elderly patients with recent and previous strokes. Ann Acad Med Singapore. 2003;32:790–4.
9. Gottlieb D, Kipnis M, Sister E, Vardi Y, Brill S. Validation of the 50 ml3 drinking test for evaluation of post-stroke dysphagia. Disabil Rehabil. 1996;18:529–32.
10. Hind NP, Wiles CM. Assessment of swallowing and referral to speech and language therapists in acute stroke. Q J Med. 1998;91:829–35.
11. Lim SH, Lieu PK, Phua SY, Seshadri R, Venketasubramanian N, Lee SH, Choo PW. Accuracy of bedside clinical methods compared with fiberoptic endoscopic examination of swallowing (FEES) in determining the risk of aspiration in acute stroke patients. Dysphagia. 2001;16:1–6.
12. Mari F, Matei M, Ceravolo MG, Pisani A, Montesi A, Provinciali L. Predictive value of clinical indices in detecting aspiration in patients with neurological disorders. J Neurol Neurosurg Psychiatry. 1997; 63:456–60.
13. McCullough GH, Rosenbek JC, Wertz RT, McCoy S, Mann G, McCullough K. Utlility of clinical swallowing examination measures

for detecting aspiration post- stroke. J Speech Lang Hear Res. 2005;48:1280–93.

14. McCullough GH, Wertz RT, Rosenbek JC, Mills RH. Inter- and intra-judge reliability of a clinical examination of swallowing in adults. Dysphagia. 2000;15:58–67.

15. Miyazaki Y, Arakawa M, Kizu J. Introduction of simple swallowing ability test for prevention of aspiration pneumonia in the elderly and investigation of factors of swallowing disorders. Yakugaku Zasshi. 2002;122:97–105.

16. Nishiwaki K, Tsuji T, Liu M, Hase K, Tanaka N, Fujiwara T. Identification of a simple screening tool for dysphagia in patients with stroke using factor analysis of multiple dysphagia variables. J Rehabil Med. 2005;37:247–51.

17. Rosenbek JC, McCullough GH, Wertz RT. Is the information about a test important? Applying the methods of evidence-based medicine to the clinical examination of swallowing. J Commun Disord. 2004;37:437–50.

18. Teramoto S, Fukuchi Y. Detection of aspiration and swallowing disorder in older stroke patients: simple swallowing provocation test versus water swallowing test. Arch Phys Med Rehabil. 2000;1:1517–9.

19. Tohara H, Saitoh E, Mays KA, Kuhlmeier K, Palmer JB. Three tests for predicting aspiration without videofluorography. Dysphagia. 2003;18:126–34.

20. Wu MC, Chang YC, Wang TG, Lin LC. Evaluating swallowing dysfunction using a 100-ml water swallowing test. Dysphagia. 2004; 19:43–7.

21. Langmore SE, Schatz K, Olsen N. Fiberoptic endoscopic examination of swallowing safety: a new procedure. Dysphagia. 1988;2:216–9.

22. Langmore SE, Schatz K, Olsen N. Endoscopic and videofluoroscopic evaluations of swallowing and aspiration. Ann Otol Rhinol Laryngol. 1991;100:678–81.

23. Leder SB, Ross DA, Briskin KB, Sasaki CT. A prospective, double-blind, randomized study on the use of topical anesthetic, vasoconstrictor, and placebo during transnasal flexible fiberoptic endoscopy. J Speech Lang Hear Res. 1997;40:1352–7.

24. Leder SB, Acton LM, Lisitano HL, Murray JT. Fiberoptic endoscopic evaluation of swallowing with and without blue-dyed food. Dysphagia. 2005;20:157–62.

25. Logemann JA. Evaluation and treatment of swallowing disorders. 2nd ed. Austin, TX: Pro-Ed; 1998.

26. Leder SB, Sasaki CT, Burrell MI. Fiberoptic endoscopic evaluation of dysphagia to identify silent aspiration. Dysphagia. 1998;13:19–21.

27. Suiter DM, Sloggy J, Leder SB. Validation of the Yale swallow protocol: a prospective double-blinded videofluoroscopic study. Dysphagia. 2014;29:199–203.

Chapter 5
Development of a Protocol: Why You Need More Than Just an Isolated 3-Ounce Water Swallow Challenge

Swallow screening appears simple but is fraught with danger. It is not acceptable to think that drinking 3 ounces of water in isolation will provide the clinician with enough information to make an informed and appropriate decision about aspiration risk status and diet recommendations. One must evaluate each patient individually to determine their unique strengths and deficits. Only then can the dysphagia specialist confidently analyze and then synthesize findings on a patient-by-patient basis to provide optimal, safe, and correct oral diet recommendations. With that being said, two additional components of the Yale Swallow Protocol are a brief cognitive evaluation and an oral mechanism examination.

Leder SB, Suiter DM, Warner HL. Answering orientation questions and following single step verbal commands: Effect on aspiration status. Dysphagia 2009;24:290–5. (Used and modified with kind permission from Springer Science + Business Media)

Can a Brief Cognitive Examination Contribute to the Assessment of Odds of Aspiration?

Objectives: In the acute care setting patients with altered mental status from such diverse etiologies as stroke, traumatic brain injury, degenerative neurological impairments, dementia, or alcohol and drug abuse are routinely referred for aspiration risk assessment. A screening protocol was developed that began with a scripted conversation between clinician and patient. Originally used to establish rapport prior to testing, a secondary goal was to determine patient orientation status and ability to follow single-step verbal commands. It would be beneficial to ascertain if this information on mental status was predictive of aspiration as documented by the criterion standard FEES. The purpose of this investigation was to determine if there was a change in risk for aspiration based upon correctly answering orientation questions, i.e., (1) What is your name? (2) Where are you right now? and (3) What year is it?, and following single-step verbal commands, i.e., (1) Open your mouth, (2) Stick out your tongue, and (3) Smile.

Methods: In a retrospective manner data were analyzed from 4,102 consecutive participants previously accrued prospectively between December 1, 1999 and January 1, 2007. Inclusion criteria were objective testing with FEES to determine aspiration status and on minimum response levels from two subscales of The Comprehensive Level of Consciousness Scale [1].

Results: The odds ratio (OR) of liquid aspiration was significantly greater ($p < 0.001$) for participants not oriented to person, place, and time (OR = 1.295, 95 % CI = 1.127–1.489). The odds ratio of liquid aspiration (OR = 1.546, 95 % CI = 1.292–1.849); puree aspiration (OR = 1.480, 95 % CI = 1.201–1.823); and being deemed unsafe for any oral intake (OR = 1.663, 95 % CI = 1.368–2.022) were significantly greater ($p < 0.001$) for participants unable to follow single-step verbal commands.

Conclusions: Answering orientation questions and following single-step verbal commands provides information on prediction of aspiration risk for liquid and puree food consistencies as well as overall eating status *prior to* swallowing assessment. Clinical knowledge of potential increased risk of aspiration allows for optimization of swallowing success.

Keywords: Deglutition, Deglutition disorders, Cognition, Screening, Aspiration risk, Oral alimentation

Introduction

The practice of evidence-based medicine integrates individual clinical experience with the best available external clinical evidence from systematic research [2]. Patients with altered mental status are routinely referred for swallow screening. These patients have diverse etiologies such as stroke, traumatic brain injury, degenerative neurological impairments, dementia, or alcohol and drug abuse. Various orientation questions and verbal commands have been used as part of the screening process for aspiration risk and a correlation was reported between cognitive problems and dysphagia in both stroke patients [3, 4] and adult patients referred for dysphagia testing [5].

A swallow screening protocol that began with a scripted conversation between clinician and patient to determine orientation status and ability to follow single-step verbal commands was employed. The goals were to establish rapport prior to testing while simultaneously collecting information for a general impression of basic cognitive functioning. It was not known, however, if this routinely collected information pertaining to mental status could also contribute to a priori knowledge of aspiration status based on objective FEES results. This is especially important in the acute care setting since patients' medical conditions often change rapidly, e.g., after antibiotic therapy or adequate hydration, as do their functional skills, e.g., ability and motivation to participate in rehabilitation, and mental status, e.g., improved alertness in recovery after stroke, traumatic brain injury, or alcohol and drug withdrawal [6]. Therefore, the clinician can potentially be alerted to a change in the risk for aspiration if orientation and/or command following change from correct to incorrect or vice versa.

It would be of interest to determine and beneficial to know if answering specific orientation questions and following specific single-step verbal commands are predictive of aspiration status *prior to* screening for aspiration risk in a large and heterogeneous population sample. The purpose of this investigation was to determine the risk for aspiration using the criterion standard FEES based upon correctly answering orientation questions, i.e.,

TABLE 5.1.   Participant demographic information.

Gender[a]	Males	Females
	$N=2,314$ (56.5 %)	$N=1,780$ (43.5 %)
Age[b]	$\overline{X}=66.3$ year	$\overline{X}=70.3$ year
	(Range = 2.0–105.0 year)	(Range = 2.0–105.0 year)

With kind permission from Springer Science+Business Media: Leder SB, Suiter DM, Warner HL. Answering orientation questions and following single step verbal commands: Effect on aspiration status. Dysphagia 24:290–295, 2009
[a]Missing data for 8 (0.2 %) participants
[b]Missing data for 20 (0.5 %) participants

(1) What is your name? (2) Where are you right now? and (3) What year is it?, and following single step verbal commands, i.e., (1) Open your mouth, (2) Stick out your tongue, and (3) Smile.

Data from a total of 4,102 inpatients (32 subjects have been added to the original study) from a large, urban, tertiary care, teaching hospital were collected and analyzed. There were 2,314 males (age range 2–105 year, mean 66 year) and 1,780 females (age range 2–105 year, mean 70 year). Table 5.1 shows participant demographics, Table 5.2 shows participant diagnostic categories, and Fig. 5.1 shows number of participants by age.

Inclusion criteria for candidacy for a swallow evaluation were based on specific minimum levels from two subscales of The Comprehensive Level of Consciousness Scale [1]. This scale provided detailed and reliable information for the assessment of acute and severe impairments of neurological functioning. General Responsiveness (Scale 7, Item #8) was defined as the person is fully aroused and alert or, if asleep, arouses and attends to the examiner following only mild or moderate stimulation. The arousal outlasts the duration of the stimulus. Best communicative effort (Scale 8, Item #3) was defined as the person visually tracks an object passed through his/her visual field and/or turns his/her head toward the examiner as if wishing to communicate or the patient generates spontaneous moaning or muttering with reliable eye contact or searching behaviors.

Prior to FEES testing, each participant was asked: (1) What is your name? (2) Where are you right now? and (3) What year is it? Each participant was then given the verbal commands to: (1) Open your mouth, (2) Stick out your tongue, and (3) Smile. The correctness of all three orientation questions and all three

TABLE 5.2.   Participant diagnostic categories.

Diagnostic category	Number
Cardiothoracic surgery	220
Esophageal surgery	78
Head and Neck surgery	172
Neurosurgery	317
Medical	821
Pulmonary	642
Cancer	168
Other medical	412
Left stroke	302
Right stroke	262
Brainstem stroke	54
Parkinson's disease	30
Dementia	127
Other neurological	497
Total	4,102

With kind permission from Springer Science + Business Media: Leder SB, Suiter DM, Warner HL. Answering orientation questions and following single step verbal commands: Effect on aspiration status. Dysphagia 24:290–295, 2009

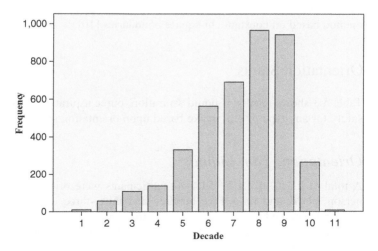

FIG. 5.1.   Age distribution of participants. (With kind permission from Springer Science + Business Media: Leder SB, Suiter DM, Warner HL. Answering orientation questions and following single step verbal commands: Effect on aspiration status. Dysphagia 24:290–295, 2009).

commands were recorded. Stimuli were given orally in English or Spanish as appropriate.

FEES testing consisted of three boluses of puree consistency (yellow pudding) followed by three liquid boluses (white milk), as these colors have excellent contrast with pharyngeal and laryngeal mucosa [7]. The standard FEES protocol as described in Chap. 3 was followed. Aspiration was defined as entry of material into the airway below the level of the true vocal folds [8] and silent aspiration occurred when there were no external behavioral signs such as coughing or choking [9]. Aspiration on a single trial constituted identification of aspiration. A safe swallow was defined as no aspiration and an unsafe swallow was defined as aspiration of both liquid and puree consistencies during FEES.

FEES outcomes were the criteria references to which orientation and command following were compared. Two-by-two contingency tables were developed to compare rates of liquid aspiration, puree aspiration, and safe or unsafe swallowing relative to orientation status and command following ability. Due to the retrospective nature of the study design, Pearson's chi-square tests and odds ratios (OR) were then computed to determine aspiration risk. Confidence intervals for odds ratios were computed by a general method based on constant chi-square boundaries [10].

Orientation Status

Table 5.3 shows results of liquid aspiration, puree aspiration, and safety for any type of oral intake based upon orientation status.

Orientation: Thin Liquids

A total of 2,230 of 4,102 (54.4 %) participants were oriented to person, place, and time. Five hundred and thirty-three of 2,230 (23.9 %) aspirated thin liquids during instrumental assessment and 1,697 (76.1 %) did not. A total of 1,872 of 4,102 (45.6 %) participants were not oriented and 542 (29.0 %) aspirated thin liquids during instrumental assessment and 1,330 (71.0 %) did not.

TABLE 5.3.   Results of liquid aspiration, puree aspiration, and safety for any type of oral intake based upon orientation status.

Aspiration status	Orientation to person, place, and time		Total
	Yes (%)	No (%)	
Liquid aspiration[a]			
Yes	533 (23.9)	542 (29.0)	1,075
No	1,697 (76.1)	1,330 (71.0)	3,027
Total	2,230	1,872	4,102
Puree aspiration			
Yes	352 (15.8)	318 (17.0)	670
No	1,878 (84.2)	1,554 (83.0)	3,432
Total	2,230	1,872	4,102
Safe for oral intake			
Yes	1,833 (82.2)	1,499 (80.0)	3,330
No	397 (17.8)	373 (20.0)	770
Total	2,230	1,872	4,102

With kind permission from Springer Science + Business Media: Leder SB, Suiter DM, Warner HL. Answering orientation questions and following single step verbal commands: Effect on aspiration status. Dysphagia 24:290–295, 2009
[a]$p < 0.001$

Pearson's chi-square results revealed a significant association between orientation and aspiration status (χ^2 [1, N = 4,102] = 13.230, $p \leq 0.001$). Odds ratio of liquid aspiration was significantly greater for individuals not oriented to person, place, and time than for individuals who were oriented (OR = 1.295, 95 % CI = 1.127–1.489).

Orientation: Puree

Three hundred and fifty-two of 2,230 (15.8 %) participants who were oriented to person, place, and time aspirated puree during instrumental assessment and 1,878 (84.2 %) did not. Three hundred and eighteen of 1,872 (17.0 %) participants who were not oriented aspirated puree during instrumental assessment and 1,554 (83 %) did not. Pearson's chi-square results were nonsignificant ($p > 0.05$). Odds ratio risk of puree aspiration was not significantly greater for individuals who were not oriented than for those who were (OR = 1.093, 95 % CI = 0.926–1.290).

Orientation: Oral Intake

A total of 397 of 2,230 (17.8 %) participants who were oriented to person, place, and time were deemed unsafe for oral intake and a total of 373 of 1,872 (20.0 %) participants who were not oriented were deemed unsafe for oral intake. Pearson's chi-square results were nonsignificant ($p > 0.05$). Odds ratio risk of being deemed potentially unsafe for any oral intake did not significantly differ based upon orientation status (OR = 1.150, 95 % CI = 0.983–1.345).

Command Following

Table 5.4 shows results of liquid aspiration, puree aspiration, and safety for any type of oral intake based upon ability to follow single one-step verbal commands.

TABLE 5.4.   Results of liquid aspiration, puree aspiration, and safety for any type of oral intake based upon ability to follow single-step verbal commands.

	Follow single-step verbal commands		
Aspiration status	Yes (%)	No (%)	Total
Liquid aspiration[a]			
Yes	853 (24.8)	221 (33.7)	1,074
No	2,589 (75.2)	434 (66.3)	3,023
Total	3,442	655	4,097[b]
Puree aspiration[a]			
Yes	531 (15.4)	139 (21.2)	670
No	2,911 (84.6)	516 (78.8)	3,427
Total	3,442	655	4,097[b]
Safe for oral intake[a]			
Yes	2,842 (82.6)	485 (74.0)	3,327
No	600 (17.4)	170 (26.0)	770
Total	3,442	655	4,097[b]

With kind permission from Springer Science + Business Media: Leder SB, Suiter DM, Warner HL. Answering orientation questions and following single step verbal commands: Effect on aspiration status. Dysphagia 24:290–295, 2009
[a] $p < 0.001$
[b] Missing data for 5 (0.1 %) participants

Command Following: Thin Liquids

A total of 3,442 of 4,097 (84.0 %) participants were able to follow one-step commands (data are missing for 5 participants). Eight hundred and fifty-three of 3,442 (24.8 %) aspirated thin liquids during instrumental assessment and 2,589 (75.2 %) did not. A total of 655 of 4,097 (16.0 %) participants were unable to follow commands and 221 (33.7 %) aspirated thin liquids during instrumental assessment and 434 (66.3 %) did not. Pearson's chi-square analysis revealed a significant association between ability to follow commands and liquid aspiration status (χ^2 [1, $N=4{,}097$]$=22.831$, $p \leq 0.001$). Odds ratio risk of liquid aspiration was significantly greater for participants who were unable to follow single commands than for those able to follow single commands (OR = 1.546, 95 % CI = 1.292–1.849).

Command Following: Puree

Five hundred and thirty-one of 3,442 (15.4 %) participants who were able to follow commands aspirated puree during instrumental assessment and 2,911 (84.6 %) did not. One hundred and thirty-nine of 655 (21.2 %) participants who were unable to follow commands aspirated puree during instrumental assessment and 516 (78.8 %) did not. Pearson's chi-square analysis revealed a significant relationship between command following ability and puree aspiration status (χ^2 [1, $N=4{,}097$]$=13.638$, $p \leq 0.001$). Odds ratio risk of puree aspiration was significantly greater for participants who were unable to follow single commands than for those able to follow single commands (OR = 1.480, 95 % CI = 1.201–1.823).

Command Following: Oral Intake

Six hundred of 3,442 (17.4 %) participants who were able to follow commands were deemed unsafe for oral intake and 170 of 655 (26.0 %) participants who were unable to follow commands were deemed unsafe for oral intake. Pearson's chi-square analysis revealed a significant association between command following ability and oral intake status (χ^2 [1, N=4,097]=26.356, $p \leq 0.001$). Odds ratio risk of being deemed unsafe for any oral intake was significantly greater for participants who were unable to follow single commands than for those able to follow single commands (OR=1.663, 95 % CI=1.368–2.022).

Clinical Importance

It is advantageous to test for orientation and command following *prior to swallow screening*. These quick and easy assessments allow for the establishment of clinician–patient rapport while simultaneously providing valuable clinical information on the risk of aspiration on the upcoming screen or dysphagia evaluation. Specifically, knowledge of this information informs the clinician that if the patient is not oriented to person, place, and time then the risk of aspiration with thin liquids is significantly greater than if oriented. Similarly, if the patient cannot follow commands the clinician should be aware that the risk of aspiration with both thin liquids and puree as well as the potential of being deemed unsafe for any type of oral intake is significantly greater than if command following is successful.

Knowledge of potential increased risk of aspiration prior to swallow screening or dysphagia testing is of direct clinical benefit. The clinical importance of research findings is based upon how data are used in the clinical setting. The fact that a given patient cannot answer orientation questions or follow single-step verbal commands should alert the clinician to potential increased aspiration risk. It does not mean that screening should be deferred but rather extra care taken during administration and interpretation of the Yale Swallow Protocol. For example, if a patient is not oriented or is unable to follow commands consistently but nevertheless passes the protocol, the clinician must recommend appropriate feeding strategies in order to promote successful resumption of oral alimentation. Such strategies include 1:1 supervision at mealtimes, assistance with feeding, cutting solid food into smaller pieces, and limiting drinking to single small (5–10 cc) bolus volumes.

Although clinicians may be using other questions and commands [3, 4], the exemplars used in the present study are based on systematic research and satisfy the requirements of evidence-based medicine [2]. In addition, more patients aspirated thin liquids than puree consistencies in the present study. This finding corroborates earlier reports of increased frequency of thin liquid aspiration during dysphagia testing [11, 12]. Therefore, if orientation and command following are impaired the clinician should be aware that the potential risk of liquid aspiration for that particular patient is increased significantly. In this case, a screening protocol or instrumental dysphagia evaluation that starts with thin liquids should be modified to begin with puree consistency which has the potential to be swallowed more successfully. All of the above efforts are implemented on an individual basis to reduce the potential risk of aspiration in order to achieve the most beneficial swallowing outcome.

Conclusions

In conclusion, the more knowledge a clinician has prior to either a swallow screen or instrumental evaluation the better the patient care will be. Extra care can then be taken for those patients when a priori knowledge of potential increased risk of aspiration for thin liquid and/or puree food consistencies is present. Ascertaining the potential risk of aspiration and potential for safe oral intake *prior to testing* allows for a more individualized evaluation.

It is important to note, however, that information obtained from the brief cognitive screen [13] and the oral mechanism examination [14], discussed below, provides information only on odds of aspiration risk with the 3-ounce water swallow challenge and should not necessarily be used as exclusionary criteria for administering the Yale Swallow Protocol. In other words, there will be patients who do poorly on the cognitive and oral mechanism parts of the protocol but nonetheless are able to successfully drink 3 ounces of water. These patients can be ordered an oral diet with specific recommendations to promote as safe swallowing as possible.

Leder SB, Suiter DM, Murray J, Rademaker AW. Can an oral mechanism examination contribute to the assessment of odds of aspiration? Dysphagia 2013;28:370–5. (Used and modified with kind permission from Springer Science + Business Media)

Can an Oral Mechanism Examination Contribute to the Assessment of Odds of Aspiration?

Objectives: Use of an oral mechanism examination by speech-language pathologists is ubiquitous and long-standing despite a paucity of research supporting its clinical utility in dysphagia diagnostics. The purpose of this study was to investigate if components of an oral mechanism examination, i.e., binary judgments (complete/incomplete) of labial closure, lingual range of motion, and facial symmetry, were associated with increased odds of aspiration as confirmed by subsequent instrumental testing.

Methods: Study design was a single group consecutively referred case series with a single judge. A total of 4,102 consecutive inpatients from a large, urban, tertiary care teaching hospital were accrued, with 3,919 meeting the inclusion criterion of adequate cognitive ability to participate in an oral mechanism examination followed immediately by FEES.

Results: Stepwise multiple logistic regression analysis indicated that participants with incomplete lingual range of motion had an odds of aspiration that was 2.72 times the odds of aspiration in those with complete lingual range of motion (95 % confidence interval 1.96–3.79, $p < 0.0001$) and incomplete lingual range of motion was an independent risk factor for aspiration regardless of labial closure and facial symmetry. Participants with incomplete facial symmetry had an odds of aspiration that was 0.76 times the odds of aspiration in those with complete facial symmetry (95 % confidence interval 0.61–0.95, $p = 0.017$). Isolated incomplete labial closure did not affect the odds of aspiration ($p > 0.05$).

Conclusions: New and clinically relevant information was found for lingual range of motion and facial symmetry, i.e., when incomplete the clinician should be alerted to potential increased odds of aspiration during subsequent instrumental dysphagia testing.

Keywords: Deglutition, Deglutition disorders, Oral mechanism, Screening, Aspiration risk, Oral alimentation

Introduction

Use of an oral mechanism examination by speech-language pathologists is ubiquitous and long-standing in dysphagia diagnostics despite a paucity of research regarding its clinical utility. Specifically, there are scant publications in support of the premise that results of an oral mechanism examination are useful specific to subsequent instrumentally confirmed aspiration events. A call for research to address the importance of oral motor abilities as a component of comprehensive dysphagia assessment was made in 1999 [15], but very little subsequent research on adverse events, such as aspiration, has been published based upon results of an oral mechanism examination.

All research, to date, that included an oral mechanism examination during clinical dysphagia screening to determine potential aspiration risk used confirmatory videofluoroscopic testing. Logemann et al. [16] included facial droop in the screening procedure but made no mention of labial closure or lingual mobility. McCullough [4, 17, 18] included tongue (side to side) and lip (pucker/retract) movements during clinical assessment but did not include facial symmetry.

It would be of interest to determine how information obtained from an oral mechanism examination contributes to the dysphagia specialist's knowledge of odds of aspiration prior to instrumental evaluation. The purpose of this study was to investigate if components of an oral mechanism examination, i.e., binary (complete/incomplete) judgments of labial closure, lingual range of motion, and facial symmetry, were associated with increased odds of aspiration as confirmed by subsequent instrumental testing.

A total of 4,102 consecutive inpatients referred between January 1, 2000 and December 31, 2007 to speech-language pathology for swallowing testing by their attending physician, physician assistant, or advanced practice nurse practitioner participated. Inclusion criterion was adequate cognitive ability [13] to participate in an oral mechanism examination. A total of 3,919 participants who met the study criterion first received an oral mechanism examination followed immediately by FEES. Table 5.5 shows participant demographics and Table 5.6 shows participant diagnostic categories at time of hospital admission.

TABLE 5.5.   Participant demographics.

Gender[a]	
Females	$N=1,780$ (43.5 %)
Males	$N=2,314$ (56.5 %)
Age[b]	
Females	$\bar{X}=70.30$ years (range$=2.0$–105.0 years)
Males	$\bar{X}=66.27$ years (range$=2.2$–105.0 years)

With kind permission from Springer Science+Business Media:
Leder SB, Suiter DM, Murray J, Rademaker AW. Can an oral
mechanism examination contribute to the assessment of odds of
aspiration? Dysphagia 28;370–374, 2013
[a]Data are missing for 8 (0.2 %) participants
[b]Data are missing for 20 (0.5 % participants

TABLE 5.6.   Diagnostic categories at time of admission.

Diagnostic category	Participants[a]
Cancer	168
Cardiothoracic surgery	220
Dementia	127
Esophageal surgery	78
Head and Neck surgery	172
Medical	1,214
Neurological (traumatic brain injury/other)	497
Neurosurgery	317
Parkinson's disease	30
Pulmonary	642
Stroke (left hemisphere)	302
Stroke (right hemisphere)	262
Stroke (brainstem)	54

With kind permission from Springer Science+Business Media: Leder SB,
Suiter DM, Murray J, Rademaker AW. Can an oral mechanism examination
contribute to the assessment of odds of aspiration? Dysphagia 28;370–374, 2013
[a]Missing data for 183 (4.5 %) participants due to inadequate cognitive ability to
participate in the oral mechanism examination

All participants first had an oral mechanism examination to determine if labial closure, lingual range of motion, and facial symmetry were either complete or incomplete. The operational definitions were as follows: (1) Labial closure was the ability to close the lips completely with no observable gaps; (2) Lingual range of motion was the ability to protrude the tongue anteriorly beyond the lips and lateralize to the right and left labial commissures; and (3) Facial symmetry was the ability to smile and pucker symmetrically. Instructions were given verbally with visual demonstration as necessary.

FEES testing consisted of three boluses of puree consistency (yellow pudding) followed by three liquid boluses (white milk), as these colors have excellent contrast with pharyngeal and laryngeal mucosa [7]. The standard FEES protocol as described in Chap. 3 was followed. Aspiration was defined as entry of material into the airway below the level of the true vocal folds [8]) and silent aspiration occurred when there were no external behavioral signs such as coughing or choking [9]. Aspiration on a single trial constituted identification of aspiration. A safe swallow was defined as no aspiration and an unsafe swallow was defined as aspiration of both liquid and puree consistencies during FEES.

Reliability Testing

All oral mechanism and FEES examinations were judged live. A 100 % non-blinded agreement between the endoscopist (SBL) and assisting health-care professional, e.g., physician, physician assistant, speech-language pathologist, registered nurse, or respiratory therapist, was required to confirm both oral mechanism functioning and tracheal aspiration. Confirmatory inter-rater reliability for the oral mechanism examination was performed with 25 additional participants. Experienced speech-language pathologists as well as naïve physician assistants, registered nurses, physical therapists, and occupational therapists participated. There were a total of 228 blinded and independent ratings, i.e., 76 each for lingual range of motion, labial closure, and facial symmetry. Inter-rater agreement was 100 % for binary (complete/incomplete) judgments of labial closure, lingual range of motion, and facial symmetry.

Confirmatory intra- and inter-rater agreement of FEES findings was performed with 128 additional participants. Two speech-language pathologists and one otolaryngologist experienced in interpreting FEES results independently and blindly reviewed the swallows on a digital swallowing workstation. Using real-time

TABLE 5.7.   Univariate analyses of incidences of aspiration associated with complete/incomplete labial closure, lingual range of motion, and facial symmetry.

	Incidence of aspiration (%)
Labial closure	
Complete	851/3,747 (22.7 %)
Incomplete	49/172 (28.5 %)
Odds Ratio = 1.36 (95 % CI 0.97–1.90), $p = 0.08$	
Lingual range of motion	
Complete	823/3,740 (22.1 %)
Incomplete	72/179 (40.2 %)
Odds Ratio = 2.37 (95 % CI 0.76–1.14), $p < 0.0001$	
Facial symmetry	
Complete	760/3,281 (23.2 %)
Incomplete	140/638 (21.9 %)
Odds Ratio = 0.93 (95 % CI 0.76–1.14), $p = 0.50$	

With kind permission from Springer Science + Business Media: Leder SB, Suiter DM, Murray J, Rademaker AW. Can an oral mechanism examination contribute to the assessment of odds of aspiration? Dysphagia 28;370–374, 2013

analysis with repeat viewing as needed, both intra- and inter-rater agreement ratings were 100 % for tracheal aspiration on at least one liquid or puree swallow during FEES.

Labial Closure, Lingual Range of Motion, Facial Symmetry, and Aspiration

Of the 3,919 participants, 172 (4.4 %) exhibited incomplete labial closure, 179 (4.6 %), incomplete lingual range of motion, and 638 (16.3 %) incomplete facial symmetry. A total of 900 (23.0 %) participants aspirated during FEES testing. Table 5.7 shows univariate analyses of incidences of aspiration associated with complete/incomplete judgments of labial closure, lingual range of motion, and facial symmetry. Only incomplete lingual range of motion was significantly associated with an increased odds ratio for aspiration, i.e., 72/179 (40.2 %) versus 823/3,740 (22.1 %), odds ratio = 2.37, $p < 0.0001$.

A stepwise multiple logistic regression analysis was conducted to determine odds of aspiration for the 3,919 participants based on a binary (complete/incomplete) judgment of lip closure, lingual range of motion, and facial symmetry. Significant variables in the resulting model were lingual range of motion and facial symmetry. Odds ratios indicated that participants with incomplete lingual range of motion had an odds of aspiration that was 2.72 times the odds of aspiration in those with complete lingual range of motion (95 % confidence interval 1.96–3.79, $p < 0.0001$). Participants with incomplete facial symmetry had an odds of aspiration that was 0.76 times the odds of aspiration in those with complete facial symmetry (95 % confidence interval 0.61–0.95, $p = 0.017$). Isolated incomplete labial closure did not affect the odds of aspiration ($p > 0.05$).

It was found that when either lingual range of motion or facial symmetry is judged incomplete the clinician should be alerted to the potential for increased odds of aspiration during subsequent instrumental dysphagia testing. Further, the contribution of facial symmetry in the regression model is interesting. Univariate analysis found only incomplete lingual range of motion to be associated with odds of aspiration (Table 5.7). However, the stepwise logistic regression model found a robust 2.72 increase in odds of aspiration associated with incomplete lingual range of motion but a weak 0.76 increased odds of aspiration associated with incomplete facial symmetry. Therefore, the dysphagia specialist may choose to place increased clinical importance with regard to odds of aspiration on incomplete lingual range of motion versus incomplete facial symmetry.

Importantly, incomplete lingual range of motion was an independent risk factor for aspiration regardless of labial closure and facial symmetry. Incomplete facial symmetry was a risk factor for aspiration only if both lingual range of motion and labial closure were incomplete. Incomplete labial closure by itself did not affect the odds of aspiration.

Although labial closure was not associated with increased odds of aspiration, it is still a clinically relevant component of the oral mechanism examination and should continue to be evaluated in patients with suspected dysphagia. Complete labial closure prevents bolus loss and drooling and is crucial for a successful oral phase of swallowing. Referral to neurology or otolaryngology, to determine if a lesion or tumor, respectively, is the etiology of incomplete labial closure is appropriate. Once an etiology is determined, e.g., neurological (apraxia or paresis) or surgical (soft tissue insult or nerve resection), appropriate rehabilitation can be instituted.

It is advantageous to perform a baseline oral mechanism examination before surgery, irradiation, or chemotherapy [19]. This information is useful when counseling the patient regarding any possible new posttreatment changes in feeding skills, e.g., difficulty taking bolus off spoon or drinking with a cup/straw, and swallow function, e.g., poor oral bolus control including drooling and stasis as well as mastication changes with specific food textures.

An oral mechanism examination is also a useful method for tracking longitudinal changes in swallow function. If changes in the oral mechanism examination occur it is easy to readminister the Yale Swallow Protocol. If passed again no intervention is warranted but if failed, an appropriate referral for an instrumental swallowing evaluation, i.e., endoscopic or videofluoroscopic, with the goal of enhancing patient safety, efficiency, and quality-of-life can be made.

Conclusions

In conclusion, two components of an oral mechanism examination, i.e., incomplete lingual range of motion and incomplete facial symmetry, increased the odds of aspiration as observed during subsequent instrumental dysphagia testing. Incomplete labial closure, although not associated with increased odds of aspiration, remains an important component to evaluate. An oral mechanism examination can be used to compare pre/posttherapeutic interventions and outcomes, to document longitudinal changes in oral motor and swallowing functions, and to help determine where and when to focus therapy to improve dysphagia.

But similar to results of cognitive testing (discussed above), results obtained from the oral mechanism examination [13] provide information only on odds of aspiration risk with the 3-ounce water swallow challenge and should not necessarily be used as exclusionary criteria for administering the Yale Swallow Protocol. Again, there will be patients who do poorly on the cognitive and oral mechanism parts of the protocol but nonetheless successfully drink 3 ounces of water. These patients can be ordered an oral diet with specific recommendations to promote as safe swallowing as possible.

References

1. Stanczak DE, White JG, Gouview WD, Moehle KA, Daniel M, Novack T, Long CJ. Assessment of level of consciousness following severe neurological insult: a comparison of the psychometric qualities of the Glasgow coma scale and the comprehensive level of consciousness scale. J Neurosurg. 1984;60:955–60.
2. Sackett DL. Evidence based research: what it is and what it isn't. BMJ. 1996;312:71–2.
3. Barer DH. The natural history and functional consequences of dysphagia after hemispheric stroke. J Neurol Neurosurg Psychiatry. 1989;52:236–41.
4. McCullough GH, Rosenbek JC, Wertz RT, McCoy S, Mann G, McCullough K. Utility of clinical swallowing measures for detecting aspiration post-stroke. J Speech Lang Hear Res. 2005;48:1280–93.
5. Martin BJW, Curlew MM. The incidence of communication disorders in dysphagic patients. J Speech Hear Dis. 1990;55:28–32.
6. Leder SB. Serial fiberoptic endoscopic swallowing evaluations in the management of patients with dysphagia. Arch Phys Med Rehabil. 1998;79:1264–9.
7. Leder SB, Acton LM, Lisitano HL, Murray JT. Fiberoptic endoscopic evaluation of swallowing with and without blue-dyed food. Dysphagia. 2005;20:157–62.
8. Logemann JA. Evaluation and treatment of swallowing disorders. 2nd ed. Austin, TX: Pro-Ed; 1998.
9. Leder SB, Sasaki CT, Burrell MI. Fiberoptic endoscopic evaluation of dysphagia to identify silent aspiration. Dysphagia. 1998;13:19–21.
10. Fleiss JL. Statistical methods for rates and proportions. 2nd ed. New York, NY: Wiley; 1981. Section 5.6.
11. Feinberg MJ, Knebl J, Tully J, Segall L. Aspiration and the elderly. Dysphagia. 1990;5:61–71.
12. Kuhlemeier KV, Palmer JB, Rosenberg D. Effect of liquid bolus consistency and delivery method on aspiration and pharyngeal retention in dysphagia patients. Dysphagia. 2001;16:119–22.
13. Leder SB, Suiter DM, Warner HL. Answering orientation questions and following single-step verbal commands: effect on aspiration status. Dysphagia. 2009;24:290–5.
14. Leder SB, Suiter DM, Murray J, Rademaker AW. Can an oral mechanism examination contribute to the assessment of odds of aspiration? Dysphagia. 2013;28:370–4.

15. McCullough GH, Wertz RT, Rosenbek JC, Dinneen C. Clinician's preferences and practices in conducting clinical/bedside and videofluoroscopic examinations of swallowing. Am J Speech Lang Path. 1999;8:149–63.
16. Logemann JA, Veis S, Colangelo L. A screening procedure for oropharyngeal dysphagia. Dysphagia. 1999;14:44–51.
17. McCullough GH, Wertz RT, Rosenbek JC, Mills RH, Ross KB, Ashford JR. Inter- and intrajudge reliability of a clinical examination of swallowing in adults. Dysphagia. 2000;15:58–67.
18. McCullough GH, Wertz RT, Rosenbek JC. Sensitivity and specificity of clinical/bedside signs for detecting aspiration in adults subsequent to stroke. J Commun Disord. 2001;34:55–72.
19. Starmer HH, Gourin CG, Lua LL, Burkhead L. Pretreatment swallowing assessment in head neck cancer patients. Laryngoscope. 2011;121: 1208–11.

Chapter 6
Generalizing the Yale Swallow Protocol to Different Patient Populations: Time to Change

The majority of swallow screens have dealt with the stroke population. But why focus solely on stroke? While this is understandable because many patients exhibit swallowing problems post-stroke there is nothing inherently unique about swallowing and aspiration risk in the stroke population. Many other diagnostic categories [1], e.g., pulmonary [2], trauma [3], and geriatrics [4], present with similar and even potentially higher incidences of aspiration risk as the stroke population. In order for a swallow screening protocol to be both effective and generalizable it must be validated on and useful for all patients. This is precisely what the Yale Swallow Protocol does.

We have shown that a simple 3-ounce water swallow challenge is a useful component to use in the determination of potential aspiration risk [1]. As discussed in Chap. 5, the additional components of both a brief cognitive evaluation [5] and oral mechanism examination [6] allow for a much richer and more patient-oriented protocol. When the experienced clinician synthesizes information provided by the entire three component protocol, there is potential to improve upon the already reported high 96.5 % sensitivity, high 97.9 % negative predictive value, and low <2.0 % false negative rate found with using the isolated 3-ounce challenge.

S.B. Leder and D.M. Suiter, *The Yale Swallow Protocol: An Evidence-Based Approach to Decision Making*, DOI 10.1007/978-3-319-05113-0_6, © Springer International Publishing Switzerland 2014

Change Always Has Challenges but Challenges Can Only Be Overcome Through Change

It was time. We had to transition our evidence-based research to clinical practice. So a decision was made that after January 01, 2008 we would *not* first perform an instrumental dysphagia evaluation, neither FEES nor VFSS, on new swallow evaluation consults. *Rather we would first administer the Yale Swallow Protocol and proceed according to its recommendations.* Were we nervous? You bet we were! After all, instrumental evaluations were the standard-of-care since 1986. But we had the data to back up our convictions.

We categorized our referral populations into four broad groupings: (1) Pediatric; (2) Trauma; (3) Stroke; and (4) General Hospital. This is important because as you will see each of these groups presents with similar but different individualized needs. And remember, one of the key criteria for a successful screening tool is to have widespread applicability to virtually all potential participants.

Generalization to the Pediatric Population

Suiter DM, Leder SB, Karas DE. The 3-ounce (90 cc) water swallow challenge: A screening test for children with suspected oropharyngeal dysphagia. Otolaryngology Head & Neck Surgery 2009;140:187–90. (Used and modified with permission from SAGE Journals.)

Objectives: We wanted to investigate the clinical utility of the 3-ounce water swallow challenge to determine both aspiration status and oral feeding recommendations in children. This had never been done before in the pediatric population and if proven successful would optimize patient care.

Methods: Participants were 56 hospitalized children (age range 2–18 year; mean 13 year) referred for swallowing evaluations. All received FEES followed by the 3-ounce challenge.

Results: Twenty-two (39.3 %) participants passed and 34 (60.7 %) failed the 3-ounce challenge. Both the sensitivity and negative predictive value for predicting aspiration status during FEES as well as the sensitivity and negative predictive value for identifying individuals who were deemed safe for oral intake based on FEES results were 100 %.

Conclusions: When the 3-ounce water swallow challenge is passed, not only thin liquids but diet recommendations with puree and solid food consistencies can be made without the need for further instrumental dysphagia assessment. The 3-ounce water swallow challenge was shown to be a clinically useful component of the Yale Swallow Protocol for both identification of aspiration risk and determination of diet recommendations in children.

Keywords: Deglutition, Deglutition disorders, Pediatrics, Aspiration risk, Swallow screening, Oral alimentation

Introduction

There was no good screening test available for children referred for suspected aspiration risk. Knowledge of aspiration risk status is critically important because of the negative sequelae associated with childhood swallowing problems, e.g. failure to thrive, dehydration, oral aversion development, and pneumonia [7, 8]. Therefore, instrumental testing with either a FEES or VFSS became, by default, the first used and only reliable method to determine aspiration risk status and implement diet recommendations for children with suspected swallowing problems.

A clinically validated screen for aspiration risk in children would avoid irradiation exposure with videofluoroscopy or discomfort with trans-nasal endoscopy [9]. But such a screen had to achieve the same three goals as with adults. Specifically: (1) Determine the likelihood that aspiration risk is present; (2) Determine when to proceed to instrumental testing; and (3) Determine when it is appropriate to either begin or resume oral alimentation.

Recent research utilizing the 3-ounce water swallow challenge in a large and heterogeneous adult population sample ($n = 3,000$)

found that aspiration risk status, determination of need for instrumental testing, and safe oral diet recommendations could be made for adults. This suggests an interesting possibility for generalization to screening for suspected aspiration risk in the pediatric population. If such a benign screen was feasible, it would permit diet recommendations to be made directly in children who pass the protocol, thereby obviating irradiation exposure with VFSS or invasive testing with FEES.

The clinical question of interest is, can the 3-ounce water swallow challenge, incorporated as one of the components of the Yale Swallow Protocol, accurately identify children who are potential aspiration risks and, when passed, recommend specific oral diets without the need for further instrumental swallow testing.

Fifty-six inpatients, 33 males and 23 females, from a large, urban, tertiary care, teaching hospital were included. Patient ages ranged from 2 to 18 years (mean=13.4 year, sd=4.7 year). Participants presented with a wide variety of 14 different diagnostic categories making generalization of findings possible. Specifically, cardiothoracic surgery ($n=2$), head and neck surgery ($n=1$), neurosurgery ($n=10$), general medical ($n=8$), pulmonary ($n=2$), cancer ($n=2$), left stroke ($n=2$), right stroke ($n=1$), traumatic brain injury ($n=10$), progressive neurological disorder ($n=7$), cervical spinal cord injury ($n=3$), acute encephalopathy ($n=3$), seizure disorder ($n=1$), other neurological ($n=4$).

The methods were similar to the original adult study [1], i.e., FEES used with both thin liquid and puree food consistencies and immediately following completion of FEES each child was asked to drink 3 ounces of water.

The important and exciting information is that in children the 3-ounce challenge had 100 % sensitivity and a 100 % negative predictive value (Table 6.1). Prior to this, the only data available to support recommendations for an oral diet based on successfully passing the 3-ounce water swallow challenge was restricted to adults [1]. Therefore, avoidance of VFSS or FEES testing after passing the protocol was achieved. Since no further testing needs to be scheduled, this also allowed for more timely initiation of both oral alimentation and oral medications.

TABLE 6.1.   Sensitivity (SENS), Specificity (SPEC), Positive Predictive Value (PPV), Negative Predictive Value (NPV), Positive Likelihood Ratio (+LR) and Negative Likelihood Ratio (−LR) of the 3-Ounce Water Swallow Challenge (95 % Confidence Intervals in Parentheses) for Determining Aspiration (Asp) and Diet Recommendations.

	SENS	SPEC	PPV	NPV	+LR	−LR
Asp	100 (75–100)	51 (35–67)	38 (22–56)	100 (85–100)	2.0 (1.4–2.7)	0.00 (0.00–1.1)
Diet	100 (54–100)	44 (30–59)	18 (7–34)	100 (85–100)	1.8 (1.2–2.3)	0.00 (0.00–2.4)

Used with permission from SAGE Journals: Suiter DM, Leder SB, Karas DE. The 3-ounce (90 cc) water swallow challenge: A screening test for children with suspected oropharyngeal dysphagia. Otolaryngology Head & Neck Surgery 140:187–190, 2009

Specifically, and corroborated by FEES results, 19 of 22 (86.4 %) children who passed the 3-ounce water swallow challenge were cleared for a regular diet; 2 (9.1 %) were cleared for a soft diet; and 1 (4.5 %) was cleared for a puree diet. Similar to adult patients, diet consistency recommendations were influenced by dentition and cognitive status. Specifically, a puree diet or soft diet was recommended for patients with erupting dentition or altered mental status, and a soft or regular consistency diet was recommended for patients with adequate dentition for efficient biting and masticating. Importantly, none of the individuals who passed the water swallow challenge were subsequently made nil per os based on FEES results. That is, there were no false negatives. In addition, the efficacy of recommending oral alimentation was excellent as follow-up demonstrated that 100 % of patients successfully tolerated their oral diet.

In conclusion, the generalizability of the 3-ounce water swallow challenge has been expanded from the adult to the pediatric population. It was shown to be a clinically useful screen that when passed avoids irradiation exposure with VFSS or invasive testing with FEES, reliably determines aspiration risk, and allows for not only thin liquids but other food consistencies and oral medications to be confidently and safely recommended.

Generalization to the Adult Acute Care Population

The consequences of comorbid dysphagia in all hospitalized patients admitted with other diagnoses, derived from the 2004 to 2005 National Hospital Discharge Survey, found that a swallowing disorder was a bad prognostic indicator. Specifically, hospitalized patients 75 years or older had double the risk of dysphagia, dysphagic patients who required rehabilitation had a 13-fold increase in mortality, and dysphagia was associated with a 40 % increase in length-of-stay (2.4 vs. 4.0 days) resulting in an additional 223,027 hospitalization days per year at a staggering cost of $547,307,964 [10]. In an effort to maximize patient care and minimize costs, it is vital to determine aspiration risk status prior to recommending oral alimentation and oral medications [11] for hospitalized patients.

The following three studies dealing with trauma, stroke, and general hospital patients, respectively, continue to expand the clinical usefulness and efficacy of the Yale Swallow Protocol to different patient populations. All are based on and replicated the same sound research design and methodology [1]. Their overall goal was to demonstrate that passing the protocol allows the dysphagia specialist to proceed with an appropriate and safe oral diet without the need for further instrumental testing. As noted previously, this is important because no other swallow screen has the ability to recommend specific oral diets to patients presenting with such a wide variety of diagnostic categories. The only information other swallow screening tests can provide pertains to the patient's aspiration risk status. The next vital step of corroborating passing with instrumental testing using various food consistencies to demonstrate successful oral alimentation has not been done. After all, the ultimate goal is not just passing a screen but avoiding further instrumental swallowing testing in order to proceed directly to timely and safe recommendations for oral alimentation and oral medications. In other words, both time and money are wasted if passing a swallow screen must be followed by instrumental testing.

It is important to note that the focus of the following three investigations was *not* to determine adequacy or maintenance of nutrition and hydration following passing the protocol, but rather the protocol's effectiveness in supporting safe oral feeding based upon specific types of oral diets. Longitudinal success of diet recommendations is discussed in Chap. 11.

Generalization to Trauma Patients

Leder SB, Suiter DM, Warner HL, Kaplan LJ. Initiating safe oral feeding in critically ill intensive care and step-down unit patients based on passing a 3-ounce (90 ml) water swallow challenge. Journal of Trauma 2011;70:1203–7. (Used and modified with permission from Wolters Kluwer Health.)

Objectives: Pulmonary aspiration is a leading cause of nosocomial infection for patients in the intensive care unit (ICU) and step-down unit (SDU). A key goal is to identify patients who exhibit increased aspiration risk prior to beginning oral alimentation. This study investigated the success of recommending specific oral diets to ICU and SDU patients based on passing the Yale Swallow Protocol.

Methods: A referral-based sample of 401 ICU and 92 SDU patients were prospectively analyzed. Amount of liquid and food ingested at the next day's meal 12–24 h after passing the protocol and specific diet recommendations were accessed electronically from oral intake information entered on each participant's daily care sheets. Drinking and eating success, clinically evident aspiration events, and accuracy of diet order recommendations were recorded. Care providers were blinded to the study's purpose.

Results: All 401 ICU and 92 SDU patients were successfully drinking thin liquids and eating 12–24 h after passing the protocol. Mean volume of liquid ingested at the next day's meal was 360 cc ± 181.2 cc for ICU and 356.4 cc ± 173.5 cc for SDU patients. Percent of meal eaten ranged from 10 to 100 %. Patient care sheets indicated specific diet recommendations were followed with 100 % accuracy.

Conclusions: Successfully recommending specific oral diets for ICU and SDU patients based on passing the Yale Swallow

Protocol was supported. Importantly, when a simple bedside protocol administered by a trained provider is passed, specific diet recommendations can be made safely and confidently without the need for further instrumental dysphagia testing.

Keywords: Deglutition, Deglutition disorders, Trauma, Aspiration risk, Swallow screening, Oral alimentation

Introduction

It is neither practical nor necessary, from a resource management or clinical care perspective, to perform objective dysphagia testing on all intensive care unit (ICU) and step-down unit (SDU) patients. However, since pulmonary aspiration is a leading cause of nosocomial infection in the critically ill [12], a key goal is to identify those patients with increased aspiration risk prior to initiating oral alimentation. It is, therefore, ideal to be able to administer a validated and reliable swallowing screening test to critically ill patients before starting an oral diet. This is especially important as many patients have an a priori increased aspiration risk due to extant comorbidities and concomitant interventions including short- (<24 h) [13] or longer-term (≥24 h) endotracheal intubation [3, 14, 15], traumatic brain injury [3], other cognitive issues [16], severe deconditioning and reduced functional reserve [17], medication side effects [17], and advanced age [4, 18].

Although there is no consensus regarding the optimal type of swallowing assessment to use, the ideal clinical examination should have a sensitivity of >95 % [19] and be simple enough to be administered by a variety of qualified clinicians [20]. If such a test were universally employed, objective dysphagia testing using either endoscopy or fluoroscopy could be reserved for those patients who fail the simpler bedside swallowing screen. A protocol that incorporates a 3-ounce water swallow challenge appears to be an examination that would fit the ideal criteria outlined above.

Once the ICU or SDU patient is deemed appropriate for consideration for oral feeding, the clinician must decide on the timing of initiating oral intake and what consistency diet to prescribe. Although aspiration risk reportedly increases post-extubation [3, 14],

TABLE 6.2.   Participant characteristics from intensive care units.

Location screened	N	Gender (M/F)	Mean age (year) (standard deviation)	Age range (year)
SICU	27	13M/14F	57 (17.4)	21–93
MICU	159	90M/69F	73 (16.0)	22–101
CCU	42	23M/19F	73 (16..2)	16–95
NICU	152	76M/73F[a]	63 (16.6)	20–91
CTICU	19	11M/8F	69 (12.8)	45–88
PICU	2	1M/1F	15 (6.4)	10–19
Total	401	214M/184F	68 (17.4)	10–101

Used with permission from Wolters Kluwer Health: Leder SB, Suiter DM, Warner HL, Kaplan LJ. Initiating safe oral feeding in critically ill intensive care and step-down unit patients based on passing a 3-ounce (90 ml) water swallow challenge. Journal of Trauma 70:1203–1207, 2011
SICU Surgical, *MICU* Medical, *CICU* Cardiac, *NICU* Neurological/Neurosurgical, *CTICU* Cardio-thoracic, *PICU* Pediatric
[a]Missing gender data for three participants

patients who have never been intubated also present with comorbidities that negatively impact on swallowing success [21, 22]. It would, therefore, be highly beneficial to determine when best to initiate timely oral alimentation for recovering ICU and SDU patients in order to support the maintenance and rebuilding of lean body mass, maintain hydration, and permit the ingestion of oral medications [23]. The purpose of the present study was to investigate the success of consumption of specific oral diet recommendations to a mixed group of ICU and SDU patients based on passing the Yale Swallow Protocol.

A consecutively referred sample of 419 ICU and 100 SDU patients from a large, urban, tertiary care, teaching hospital participated. As often occurs in the acute care setting, 18 ICU and 8 SDU patients were excluded due to worsening medical, surgical, or neurological conditions necessitating nil-per-os status within 24 h after passing the protocol. Tables 6.2 and 6.3 show demographic information for ICU and SDU participants, respectively. Tables 6.4 and 6.5 show participant diagnoses grouped by ICU and SDU settings, respectively.

Patients were provided with a 3-ounce water swallow challenge with the same pass/fail criteria as in Suiter and Leder [1]. All participants were screened with the Yale Swallow Protocol.

TABLE 6.3.   Participant characteristics from step-down units.

Location screened	N	Gender M/F	Mean age (year) (standard deviation)	Age range (year)
SSDU	62	39M/23F	61 (22.3)	19–94
MSDU	7	3M/4F	73 (12.6)	52–88
CSDU	2	1M/1F	80 (17.0)	68–92
NSDU	21	14M/6F[a]	62 (18.7)	21–90
Total	92	57M/34F	63 (21.0)	19–94

Used with permission from Wolters Kluwer Health: Leder SB, Suiter DM, Warner HL, Kaplan LJ. Initiating safe oral feeding in critically ill intensive care and step-down unit patients based on passing a 3-ounce (90 ml) water swallow challenge. Journal of Trauma 70:1203–1207, 2011
SSDU Surgical, *MSDU* Medical, *CSDU* Cardiac, *NSDU* Neurological/Neurosurgical
[a]Missing gender data for 1 participant

TABLE 6.4.   Participant diagnoses grouped by intensive care unit.

Diagnosis	Intensive care unit						Total
	SICU	MICU	CICU	NICU	CTICU	PICU	
Cardiothoracic surgery	1	0	0	0	14	0	15
Esophageal surgery	1	0	1	0	0	0	2
Head and neck surgery	0	0	0	3	0	0	3
Neurosurgery	0	0	0	48	3	0	51
Medical	0	22	0	4	1	0	27
Surgery/trauma	22	0	0	0	0	0	22
Cardiac	0	0	35	0	0	0	35
Pulmonary	0	131	6	0	1	0	138
Cancer	2	1	0	3	0	0	6
Left stroke	0	0	0	29	0	0	29
Right stroke	0	1	0	26	0	1	28
Brainstem stroke	0	0	0	3	0	0	3
Other neurological	1	4	0	36	0	1	42
Total	27	159	42	152	19	2	401

Used with permission from Wolters Kluwer Health: Leder SB, Suiter DM, Warner HL, Kaplan LJ. Initiating safe oral feeding in critically ill intensive care and step-down unit patients based on passing a 3-ounce (90 ml) water swallow challenge. Journal of Trauma 70:1203–1207, 2011
SICU Surgical, *MICU* Medical, *CICU* Cardiac, *NICU* Neurological/Neurosurgical, *CTICU* Cardio-thoracic, *PICU* Pediatric

Briefly, the task requires drinking 3 ounces of water from a cup or straw, either assisted or independently, without interruption. Criteria for failure are inability to drink the entire amount, interrupted drinking, or coughing during drinking or immediately after completion.

TABLE 6.5.   Participant diagnoses grouped by step-down unit.

Diagnosis	Step-down unit				Total
	SSDU	MSDU	CSDU	NSDU	
Esophageal surgery	2	0	0	0	2
Head and neck surgery	1	0	0	0	1
Neurosurgery	0	0	0	7	7
Medical	44	5	2	1	52
Surgery/trauma	1	2	0	0	3
Cancer	5	0	0	0	5
Brainstem stroke	0	0	0	1	1
Dementia	2	0	0	1	3
Other neurological	7	0	0	11	18
Total	62	7	2	21	92

Used with permission from Wolters Kluwer Health: Leder SB, Suiter DM, Warner HL, Kaplan LJ. Initiating safe oral feeding in critically ill intensive care and step-down unit patients based on passing a 3-ounce (90 ml) water swallow challenge. Journal of Trauma 70:1203–1207, 2011
SSDU Surgical, MSDU Medical, CSDU Cardiac, NSDU Neurological/Neurosurgical

The protocol encompasses determination of the adequacy of oral motor skills for functional feeding [6], visual assessment of dentition status [6], and evaluation of basic cognitive functions such as orientation, following single verbal directions, and ability to cooperate with testing [5]. When passed, specific oral diet recommendations consisting of thin liquids with puree, soft, or regular consistency foods were then given.

Routine oral intake and diet information were recorded and accessed 12–24 h after passing the protocol on the electronic daily care sheets, and nurses were blinded to the purpose of the study. Neither the speech-language pathology nor nursing services identified any patient exhibiting overt signs of aspiration. Tables 6.6 and 6.7 show results of oral intake data collected from daily care sheets. All 401 ICU and 92 SDU study patients were successfully and safely drinking thin liquids and eating an oral diet 12–24 h after passing the protocol. The mean volume of liquid successfully ingested at the next day's meal was 360 cc ± 181.2 cc for ICU and 356.4 cc ± 173.5 cc for SDU patients. Percent of meal eaten ranged from 10 to 100 %. In addition, the daily care sheets for both ICU and SDU patients indicated that specific diet recommendations made by speech-language pathology were ordered by the physician

TABLE 6.6.   Volume (in cc) of liquid ingested at a representative meal 12–24 h after passing the 3-ounce water swallow challenge and accuracy of diet order recommendations for ICU participants.

Location screened	Volume (in cc) ingested		Mean (standard deviation)	Correct diet ordered (%)
	Minimum	Maximum		
SICU	90	640	317.3 (153.4)	100
MICU	100	1,160	340.0 (163.4)	100
CCU	60	960	340.2 (201.9)	100
NICU	60	1,280	389.3 (195.6)	100
CTICU	120	680	379.5 (166.6)	100
PICU	240	660	450.0 (297.0)	100
Totals	60	1,280	360.0 (181.2)	100

Used with permission from Wolters Kluwer Health: Leder SB, Suiter DM, Warner HL, Kaplan LJ. Initiating safe oral feeding in critically ill intensive care and step-down unit patients based on passing a 3-ounce (90 ml) water swallow challenge. Journal of Trauma 70:1203–1207, 2011
SICU Surgical, *MICU* Medical, *CICU* Cardiac, *NICU* Neurological/Neurosurgical, *CTICU* Cardio-thoracic, *PICU* Pediatric

TABLE 6.7.   Volume (in cc) of liquid ingested at a representative meal 12–24 h after passing the 3-ounce water swallow challenge and accuracy of diet order recommendations for SDU participants.

Location screened	Volume (in cc) ingested		Mean (standard deviation)	Correct diet ordered (%)
	Minimum	Maximum		
SSDU	90	980	362.4 (178.6)	100
MSDU	120	720	323.6 (192.5)	100
CSDU	100	190	145.0 (63.6)	100
NSDU	200	720	369.5 (152.5)	100
Totals	90	980	356.4 (173.5)	100

Used with permission from Wolters Kluwer Health: Leder SB, Suiter DM, Warner HL, Kaplan LJ. Initiating safe oral feeding in critically ill intensive care and step-down unit patients based on passing a 3-ounce (90 ml) water swallow challenge. Journal of Trauma 70:1203–1207, 2011
SSDU Surgical, *MSDU* Medical, *CSDU* Cardiac, *NSDU* Neurological/Neurosurgical

or licensed independent providers responsible for those patients with 100 % accuracy.

Successful oral diet recommendations for both surgical and medical ICU and SDU patients based on passing the Yale Swallow Protocol have been confirmed. Specifically, all stable ICU and SDU patients successfully drank thin liquids and ate an oral diet the day after passing. The Yale Swallow Protocol meets the criteria of a simple clinical screen that can be used by a qualified health-care professional to identify aspiration risk [20]. Perhaps most importantly, and supporting prior research [1], when the protocol is passed specific diet recommendations can be made safely and confidently without the need for further instrumental fluoroscopic or endoscopic dysphagia testing. This permits timely ingestion of oral medications, nutrition, and water [23]. In addition, confidence in the aspiration risk assessment avoids interim enteral access catheter placement while awaiting instrumental swallowing testing prior to initiating oral feeding and medications.

We recommend that if the protocol is failed, it should be repeated within 24 h. This is a reasonable approach, as ICU and SDU patients often demonstrate rapid improvement in swallowing function [5]. If subsequently passed, diet recommendations may be confidently made without the need for further dysphagia testing. If a second protocol is failed, objective endoscopic or fluoroscopic testing should be done to assess for safe oral alimentation.

A systematic review of the English literature from 1950 to 2009 ($n = 1,489$ manuscripts) from 14 electronic databases using the key words deglutition disorders, swallowing disorders, dysphagia, swallowing, and intubation identified no reliable parameters associated with an increased dysphagia and aspiration risk in critically ill patients. Specifically, age, gender, diagnosis, duration of intubation, and timing of post-extubation swallowing assessments were all *unreliable* predictors of aspiration risk [24]. Therefore, determination of an a priori aspiration risk based upon non-swallowing indicators is not supported in an evidence-based fashion. It would be appropriate, from a risk-benefit perspective, to view all ICU and SDU patients as a homogeneous group. This allows for the most important factor, identification of aspiration risk status, to be directly determined by a swallowing task.

In summary, this study supports that both surgical and medical ICU and SDU patients can be adequately assessed with regard to aspiration risk by the Yale Swallow Protocol. When the protocol was passed, and taking into consideration patient-specific factors that may influence successful oral alimentation, specific diet recommendations can be made safely and confidently without the need for further objective dysphagia testing. When administered and interpreted by a trained specialist, the Yale Swallow Protocol may be adopted as a standard bedside assessment tool both to screen ICU and SDU patients for aspiration risk and to make recommendations for initiating specific oral diets without the need for further instrumental testing.

Generalization to Stroke Patients

Leder SB, Suiter DM, Warner HL, Acton LM, Swainson BA. Success of recommending oral diets in acute stroke patients based on a 90 cc water swallow challenge protocol. Top Stroke Rehabil. 2012;19:40-4. (Used and modified with permission from Thomas Land Publishers.)

Objectives: Two of the most important issues following an acute stroke are identification of potential aspiration risk and recommendations for when to begin safe oral feeding and oral medications. This study investigated the success of recommending specific oral diet recommendations following an acute stroke based on passing the Yale Swallow Protocol.

Methods: A total of 75 acute adult stroke inpatients participated. Volume (in cc) of liquid ingested, percent of meal eaten, and specific diet recommendations made 12–24 h after passing a water swallow challenge were accessed electronically from routine oral intake information entered by nursing on each participant's daily flow sheets. Nurses were blinded to purpose of this study.

Results: All 75 participants were drinking thin liquids and eating food successfully 12–24 h after passing a 3-ounce challenge. Mean volume of liquid successfully ingested was 385.4 cc and percent of oral diet eaten ranged from 10 to 100 %. Nursing flow sheets indicated that specific diet recommendations were followed with 100 % accuracy.

Conclusions: Successfully recommending specific oral diets to acute stroke patients based on passing the protocol was supported. The Yale Swallow Protocol is an easily administered, highly reliable, cost effective, and validated clinical screen that can be used by a variety of qualified health-care professionals to identify aspiration risk. Importantly, when the protocol is passed, specific diet recommendations can be made safely and confidently without the need for further instrumental dysphagia testing.

Keywords: Deglutition, Deglutition disorders, Acute stroke, Aspiration risk, Swallow screening, Oral alimentation

Introduction

Swallowing disorders are commonly found after an acute stroke and although there is a >80 % rate of spontaneous swallowing recovery 2–4 weeks post-stroke, the greatest risk of prandial aspiration occurs during the acute post-stroke period [25, 26]. Therefore, two of the most important initial issues following an acute stroke are identification of aspiration risk and recommendations for safe oral alimentation [20] including medications [11]. It would be of great benefit to have a reliable, repeatable, evidence-based, cost-effective clinical swallow protocol with acceptable risk assessment values [27, 28] that can be administered by a variety of qualified health-care professionals in normal clinical practice to the acute stroke population [20].

As with pediatric and ICU/SDU trauma patients, it is impossible and not necessary to perform FEES or VFSS on all post-stroke patients. However, detection of eating and swallowing difficulties leading to aspiration risk must be an integral part of acute stroke management to reduce sequelae associated with unrecognized prandial aspiration [20]. It is imperative, therefore, that clinicians perform an assessment on all patients post-stroke to determine aspiration risk prior to beginning oral alimentation [29]. Instrumental videofluoroscopic or endoscopic dysphagia testing should be reserved only for those patients who fail a reliable and validated clinical swallow screen.

A large subset of stroke patients were reported in our original study [1]. Using FEES as the reference standard for determination of aspiration risk, it was found that for patients post-acute left stroke ($n = 227$) sensitivity = 97.8 % and negative predictive value = 98.8; post-acute right stroke ($n = 203$) sensitivity = 92.7 %

and negative predictive value=95.7; and post-acute brainstem stroke (n=38) sensitivity=100 % and negative predictive value=100. Importantly, when the challenge was passed success-ful diet recommendations could be made without the need for further instrumental diagnostic testing [1]. Therefore, a protocol incorporating a 3-ounce water swallow challenge component was shown to be a validated, reliable, and easily administered and interpreted tool for determination of aspiration risk that is appro-priate for use with virtually all hospitalized patients [1].

It is of great interest to determine the safety of initiating a safe oral diet as soon as possible following an acute stroke in order to prevent malnutrition and dehydration and permit ingestion of oral medications. The purpose of the present study was to investigate the success of recommending specific oral diets to patients following acute stroke based on passing the Yale Swallow Protocol.

A new cohort of 80 acute stroke patients referred for a swal-lowing study from a large, urban, tertiary care, teaching hospital participated. A total of 75 patients met the inclusion criteria of maintenance of adequate cognitive [5] and neurologic status for 12–24 h after passing the protocol (Table 6.8). Five participants (1 left hemisphere stroke, 3 right hemisphere strokes, and 1 brain-stem stroke) were excluded due to worsening cognitive and neurologic conditions, e.g., poor arousal, increased lethargy, or inability to participate with a swallowing task, which necessitated nil-per-os status within 12–24 h of passing the protocol.

TABLE 6.8.   Participant characteristics.

N	Stroke	Gender	Age	Location screened
40	Left hemisphere	24M/16F	20–91 year; $\overline{X}$=68.3[a]	Neurology ICU (N=30)
				Neurology Floor (N=10)
35	Right hemisphere	22M/13F	19–88 year; $\overline{X}$=62.9	Neurology ICU (N=29)[b]
				Neurology Floor (N=4)
5	Brainstem	3M/2	38–84 year; $\overline{X}$=65.2	Neurology ICU (N=3)
				Neurology Floor (N=2)

Used with permission from Thomas Land Publishers: Leder SB, Suiter DM, Warner HL, Acton LM, Swainson BA. Success of recommending oral diets in acute stroke patients based on a 90 cc water swallow challenge protocol. Top Stroke Rehabil. 2012;19:40–4
[a]Missing age data for 1 participant
[b]1 participant each in pediatric ICU and medical ICU

TABLE 6.9.   Volume (in cc) of liquid ingested, percent of meal eaten, and accuracy of diet recommendations made 12–24 h after passing the Yale Swallow Protocol.

| | Volume liquid ingested | | | | Percent of | |
N	Minimum	Maximum	Mean	Standard deviation	Meal eaten	Correct diet
75	120cc	1,280cc	385.cc	179.7cc	Range: 10–100 %	100 %

Used with permission from Thomas Land Publishers: Leder SB, Suiter DM, Warner HL, Acton LM, Swainson BA. Success of recommending oral diets in acute stroke patients based on a 90 cc water swallow challenge protocol. Top Stroke Rehabil. 2012;19:40-4

Methodology and procedures regarding protocol administration, data acquisition, and follow-up of diet success were identical to ICU and SDU trauma patients [30] as described previously.

Data collected from nursing oral intake daily flow sheets indicated that all 75 participants, having passed the protocol, were drinking thin liquids and eating an oral diet successfully at the 12–24 h follow-up (Table 6.9). The mean volume of liquid successfully ingested at a representative meal was 385.4 cc and percent of meal eaten ranged from 10 to 100 %. In addition, the daily flow sheets indicated that specific diet recommendations of thin liquids with puree, soft, or regular consistency foods made by speech-language pathology were being followed with 100 % accuracy. Neither speech-language pathology nor nursing identified any participant as exhibiting overt signs of aspiration during the 12–24 h follow-up period.

The present study demonstrated the success of recommending specific oral diets to acute care stroke patients based on passing the Yale Swallow Protocol. All neurologically stable acute stroke patients who passed the protocol received and drank thin liquids and ate an oral diet successfully during the 12–24 h follow-up period. The protocol meets the criteria of a simple clinical assessment that can be used by a number of qualified health-care professionals to identify aspiration risk [20], as it is easily administered, highly reliable, cost effective, and clinically validated [1]. Importantly, when the challenge is passed, aspiration risk is negligible [31] allowing for specific diet recommendations to be made safely and confidently without the need for further instrumental dysphagia testing. This permits timely ingestion of oral medications, no delay in maintaining nutrition and hydration, and with the beneficial goal of avoidance of nasogastric feeding tube placement during the acute post-stroke period.

In summary, any individual post-acute stroke may be adequately assessed with regard to potential aspiration risk by the Yale Swallow Protocol. When the protocol is passed, and taking into consideration patient specific protocol factors that may influence successful oral diet recommendations [5, 20, 29] it was reported that success rates for drinking thin liquids and eating food were 100 %. Prior supportive data specific to acute stroke patients revealed an average 96.8 % sensitivity and 97.8 % negative predictive value for correctly predicting aspiration status, and a rate of 98.5 % for successful recommendation of an oral diet [1] making the Yale Swallow Protocol a highly reliable and clinically useful swallow screen. Importantly, when administered and interpreted by a trained clinician, the protocol may be adopted as a standard bedside assessment to both determine aspiration risk and make recommendations for initiating safe and specific diet recommendations for post-acute stroke individuals without the need for further instrumental dysphagia testing.

Generalization to General Hospital Patients

Leder SB, Suiter DM, Warner HL, Acton LM, Siegel MD. Safe initiation of oral diets in hospitalized patients based on passing a 3-ounce (90 cc) water swallow challenge protocol. Q J Med 2012;105:257–63. (Used and modified with permission from Oxford University Press.)

Objectives: To determine the short-term 24-h success of recommending specific oral diets, including drinking thin liquids, to acute care hospitalized patients at risk for dysphagia based on passing the Yale Swallow Protocol.

Methods: Out of a total cohort of 1,000 participants, 907 (90.7 %) hospitalized patients met the inclusion criteria of stable medical, surgical, or neurological conditions. Specific diet recommendations and volume (in cc) of liquid ingested at the next day's meal

12–24 h after passing the protocol were accessed electronically from oral intake information entered on each participant's daily care logs. Eating and drinking success, clinically evident aspiration events, and compliance with ordering the recommended diet were recorded. Care providers were blinded to the study's purpose.

Results: All 907 patients were both eating and drinking thin liquids successfully and without overt signs of dysphagia. Median volume of liquid ingested was 340 cc (interquartile range [IQR], 240–460). Specific diet recommendations were followed with 100 % accuracy.

Conclusions: The Yale Swallow Protocol successfully identified patients who can be safely advanced to an oral diet without subsequent identification of overt signs of aspiration within 12–24 h of testing. Importantly, when the protocol administered by a trained provider is passed, specific diet recommendations, including drinking thin liquids, can be made safely and without the need for additional instrumental dysphagia testing.

Keywords: Deglutition, Deglutition disorders, Aspiration risk, Swallow screening, Oral alimentation

Introduction

Dysphagia is a sentinel symptom associated with numerous pathologies in hospitalized patients, e.g., chronic obstructive pulmonary disease [32]; stroke [33]; cardiac surgery [34]; trauma [3]; and degenerative neurologic conditions including Alzheimer's dementia [35], Parkinson's disease [36], amyotrophic lateral sclerosis [37], and multiple sclerosis [38]. Also, a longitudinal epidemiologic study reported that between 2000 and 2007 the aging of the general population resulted in dysphagia referrals doubling for 80–89 year old and tripling for 90+ year old hospitalized geriatric patients [4].

Similar to the rationale with pediatric, ICU/SDU trauma, and acute stroke patients, it is neither practical nor necessary, from both resource management and clinical care perspectives, to perform instrumental dysphagia testing with all at-risk hospitalized patients.

But since prandial pulmonary aspiration is a leading cause of nosocomial infection, a key goal is to identify those patients with increased aspiration risk prior to initiating oral alimentation [12]. It would be advantageous to administer a reliable swallow screen to all patients at risk for aspiration before starting an oral diet. This is especially important as many patients have an a priori increased aspiration risk due to extant comorbidities and concomitant interventions including, but not limited to, short- (<24 h) [13] or longer-term (≥24 h) endotracheal intubation [3, 14, 15], traumatic brain injury [3], other causes of cognitive impairment [4], severe deconditioning and reduced functional reserve [4], medication side effects [3], and advanced age [4, 18].

Once a hospitalized patient at risk for potential aspiration is deemed appropriate for consideration for oral feeding, the clinician must decide when to initiate oral intake and what diet consistency to prescribe in order to sustain safe oral alimentation to maintain and rebuild lean body mass, provide hydration, and permit the ingestion of oral medications [23]. Avoidance of prandial pulmonary aspiration as a cause of nosocomial infection is an important goal for all acute care hospitalized patients at risk for aspiration. The focus of the present study was to determine the protocol's effectiveness in determining safe oral feeding based upon specific types of oral diets. The present study investigated the success of recommending specific oral diets, including thin liquids, based on passing the Yale Swallow Protocol without the need for instrumental testing to a heterogeneous population of hospitalized patients referred for evaluation of potential aspiration risk.

Methodology and procedures regarding protocol administration, data acquisition, and follow-up of diet success were identical to our ICU/SDU trauma [30] and acute stroke studies [39].

A consecutively referred sample of 1,000 inpatients from a large, urban, tertiary care, teaching hospital participated. Table 6.10 shows demographics and Table 6.11 lists admitting diagnostic categories of all participants. A total of 907 patients participated as 93 (9.3 %) did not meet inclusion criteria either due to worsening medical, surgical, or neurological conditions necessitating nil-per-os status within 12–24 h after passing the protocol or discharge from the hospital prior to the 12–24 h follow-up period. Table 6.12 shows results of oral intake data collected from daily care logs.

TABLE 6.10. Participant characteristics.

Gender[a]	N	Median age (year) (IQR)	Age range (year)
Male	560	67 (54–79)	10–102
Female	436	70 (58–83)	14–101

Used with permission from Oxford University Press: Leder SB, Suiter DM, Warner HL, Acton LM, Siegel MD. Safe initiation of oral diets in hospitalized patients based on passing a 3-ounce (90 cc) water swallow challenge protocol. Q J Med 105:257–263, 2012
[a]Missing gender data for four participants

TABLE 6.11. Participant admitting diagnostic categories.

Diagnostic category	n	%
Medical	359	35.9
Pulmonary	210	21.0
Other neurologic	105	10.5
Neurosurgery	83	8.3
Left stroke	57	5.7
Cancer	50	5.0
Right stroke	46	4.6
Cardiothoracic surgery	24	2.4
Esophageal surgery	19	1.9
Head and neck surgery	18	1.8
Dementia	15	1.5
Brainstem stroke	9	0.9
Parkinson's disease	5	0.5
Total	1,000	100.0

Used with permission from Oxford University Press: Leder SB, Suiter DM, Warner HL, Acton LM, Siegel MD. Safe initiation of oral diets in hospitalized patients based on passing a 3-ounce (90 cc) water swallow challenge protocol. Q J Med 105:257–263, 2012

TABLE 6.12. Volume (in cc) of liquid ingested at a representative meal 12–24 h after passing the 3-ounce water swallow challenge protocol ($N=907$).

Volume (in cc) Ingested			
Minimum	Maximum	Median	IQR
50	1,280	340	240–460

Used with permission from Oxford University Press: Leder SB, Suiter DM, Warner HL, Acton LM, Siegel MD. Safe initiation of oral diets in hospitalized patients based on passing a 3-ounce (90 cc) water swallow challenge protocol. Q J Med 105:257–263, 2012

All 907 (90.7 %) study patients were drinking thin liquids successfully and safely 12–24 h after passing a 3-ounce challenge protocol.

Neither the speech-language pathology nor nursing services identified any patient as exhibiting overt signs of aspiration. The median volume of liquid successfully ingested at the next day's meal was 340.0 cc (interquartile range [IQR], 240–460). Percent of meal eaten ranged from 10 to 100 %. In addition, specific diet recommendations made by speech-language pathology were ordered by the responsible physician or licensed independent provider with 100 % accuracy. The recommended diets spanned thin liquids with puree, soft, or regular consistency foods.

Success of recommending specific oral diets for hospitalized patients based on passing the Yale Swallow Protocol has been confirmed and corroborated previous work with pediatric [40], trauma [30], and acute stroke [39] patients. Specifically, all neurologically and medically stable patients successfully drank thin liquids and ate an oral diet the day after passing the protocol. This Yale Swallow Protocol meets the criteria of a simple clinical tool that can be used by a qualified health-care professional to identify aspiration risk [20]. Most importantly and supporting our prior original research [1], when the protocol is passed specific diet recommendations can be made safely and confidently without the need for additional instrumental dysphagia testing. This permits timely ingestion of oral medications, nutrition, and water. Additionally, confidence in the swallow assessment avoids interim enteral access catheter placement while awaiting objective testing prior to initiating oral alimentation and medications.

In summary, the current study both supports and extends previous observations [30, 39, 40] of the Yale Swallow Protocols' usefulness in recommending specific oral diets to a wider range of patient diagnostic categories and supports that selected acute care hospitalized patients may be adequately assessed with regard to potential aspiration risk by the protocol. When the protocol was passed and the patient's clinical condition remained stable, specific diet recommendations, including drinking thin liquids, were made with a success rate of 100 %. When administered and interpreted by a trained specialist, data from multiple patient populations has confirmed that the Yale Swallow Protocol may be adopted as a standard clinical assessment tool to screen selected acute care hospitalized patients at risk for aspiration and, most importantly, to make recommendations for initiating specific oral diets without the need for instrumental testing.

Overall Conclusions Based on the Four Studies: Pediatrics, Trauma, Acute Stroke, and General Hospital Populations

All medically and neurologically stable patients in the four broad categories of pediatrics, trauma, acute stroke, and general hospital who passed the Yale Swallow Protocol were recommended for and successful with short-term 24-h oral alimentation. However, additional patient-specific factors should be taken into consideration. This is to ensure that ingestion of an oral diet and oral medications is safe and successful. The importance of clinical judgment and experience, in conjunction with objective information, is an essential factor in the care of the critically ill hospitalized individual with suspected increased aspiration risk.

Additional factors to consider include pre-morbid diet status; self-feeding ability or lack thereof; cognitive status, cooperativeness, and level of alertness; gross oral motor functioning; respiratory condition; endurance; and posture limitations [5, 6, 8]. All these factors need to be explored when administering and interpreting the Yale Swallow Protocol. The reason is that failure to account for these important factors may lead to an inappropriately high bedside swallow failure rate. Therefore, successful application of results entails both performing the protocol correctly (and knowing when to defer protocol administration) combined with appropriate interpretation in light of the patient's medical condition and goals of care.

For example, the clinician must be aware that patients of all ages with altered mental status, neurological impairment, traumatic brain injury, or stroke need to be evaluated and monitored at mealtimes regarding following directions, self-feeding skills, neglect, limb apraxia, nondominant upper extremity use, impulsivity, and task attentiveness. Many trauma patients in the ICU and SDU units become deconditioned and easily fatigued requiring diet modifications and assistance with feeding. All patients, especially post-acute stroke, are frustrated with their new deficits and require monitoring to determine specific diet modifications and rehabilitative needs for assistance with eating and feeding. Also, patients with swallowing problems uniformly benefit from encouragement and incremental goal updating as work toward the end goal of normal eating progresses. The dysphagia specialist, therefore, must synthesize objective, subjective, behavioral, and medical data on both an individual and continuous basis to promote safe and successful swallowing and eating.

An important caveat is that the Yale Swallow Protocol is not recommended for administration to patients who require a tracheotomy tube, e.g., for airway maintenance, ongoing mechanical ventilation, and pulmonary toilet. Silent aspiration occurs more frequently due to laryngeal desensitization from chronic aspiration of secretions [41, 42] and, in the case of head and neck cancer, the effects of combined chemo-radiation therapy [43]. Although a tracheotomy and placement of a tracheotomy tube are not causal for aspiration [21, 22], if aspiration occurs it is often silent, leading to higher false negative rates on the protocol. Instrumental testing with endoscopy or fluoroscopy is recommended for these patients. All other medical and surgical patients, however, are candidates for and will benefit from the Yale Swallow Protocol.

It is important to remember that *all* swallow assessments whether a screen or instrumental can only provide a snapshot in time of a patient's swallowing abilities. A negative test allows for safe oral alimentation only as long as the patient remains medically and neurologically stable. Careful patient monitoring after an oral diet is ordered is required because passing either a screen or instrumental test cannot guarantee continued successful swallowing behavior.

Research is presented in Chap. 11 on results of investigating longer-term follow-up for 1–5 days of eating and drinking success after passing the protocol. We acknowledge the importance of longer-term follow-up of diet recommendations based on passing the Yale Swallow Protocol. However, realities of the acute care setting, e.g., acute medical status changes, rapid discharge from general hospital beds including even direct discharge from the ICU and

SDU to extended care facilities, and billing regulations that preclude follow-up after a negative test result, justified limiting follow-up to 12–24 h in the four patient populations discussed.

References

1. Suiter DM, Leder SB. Clinical utility of the 3-ounce water swallow test. Dysphagia. 2008;23:244–50.
2. Leder SB. Incidence and type of aspiration in acute care patients requiring mechanical ventilation via a new tracheotomy. Chest. 2002;122:1721–6.
3. Leder SB, Cohn SM, Moller BA. Fiberoptic endoscopic documentation of the high incidence of aspiration following extubation in critically ill trauma patients. Dysphagia. 1998;13:208–12.
4. Leder SB, Suiter DM. An epidemiologic study on aging and dysphagia in the acute care hospitalized population: 2000–2007. Gerontology. 2009;55:714–8.
5. Leder SB, Suiter DM, Warner HL. Answering orientation questions and following single step verbal commands: effect on aspiration status. Dysphagia. 2009;24:290–5.
6. Leder SB, Suiter DM, Murray J, Rademaker AW. Can an oral mechanism examination contribute to the assessment of odds of aspiration? Dysphagia. 2013;28:370–4.
7. Martin BJ, Corlew MM, Wood H, Olson D, Golopol LA, Wingo M, Kirmani N. The association of swallowing dysfunction and aspiration pneumonia. Dysphagia. 1994;9:1–6.
8. Langmore SE, Terpenning MS, Schork A, Chen Y, Murray JT, Lopatin D, Loesche WJ. Predictors of aspiration pneumonia: how important is dysphagia? Dysphagia. 1998;13:69–81.
9. Leder SB, Karas DE. Fiberoptic endoscopic evaluation of swallowing in the pediatric population. Laryngoscope. 2000;110:1132–6.
10. Altman KW, Yu G-P, Schaefer SD. Consequence of dysphagia in the hospitalized patient. Arch Otolaryngol Head Neck Surg. 2010;136:784–9.
11. Leder SB, Lerner MZ. Nil per os except medications order in the dysphagic patient. Q J Med. 2013;106:71–5.
12. Hafner G, Neuhuber A, Hirtenfelder S, Schmedler B, Eckel H. Fiberoptic endoscopic evaluation of swallowing in intensive care unit patients. Eur Arch Otorhinolaryngol. 2008;26:441–6.
13. Heffner JE. Swallowing complications after endotracheal extubation. Chest. 2010;137:509–10.
14. de Larminat V, Montravers P, Dureil B, Desmonts JM. Alteration in swallowing reflex after extubation in intensive care unit patients. Crit Care Med. 1995;3:486–90.

15. Ajemian MS, Nirmul GB, Anderson MT, Zirlen DM, Kwasnik EM. Routine fiberoptic endoscopic evaluation of swallowing following prolonged intubation: implications for management. Arch Surg. 2001; 136:434–7.
16. Leder SB. Serial fiberoptic endoscopic swallowing examinations in the management of patients with dysphagia. Arch Phys Med Rehabil. 1998; 79:1264–9.
17. Solh A, Okada M, Bhat A, Pietrantoni C. Swallowing disorders post orotracheal intubation in the elderly. Intensive Care Med. 2003;29:1451–5.
18. Leder SB, Espinosa JF. Aspiration risk after acute stroke: comparison of clinical examination and fiberoptic endoscopic evaluation of swallowing. Dysphagia. 2002;17:214–8.
19. Ramsey DJC, Smithard DG, Kalra L. Early assessments of dysphagia and aspiration risk in acute stroke patients. Stroke. 2003;34:1252–7.
20. Leder SB, Ross DA. Investigation of the causal relationship between tracheotomy and aspiration in the acute care setting. Laryngoscope. 2000;110:641–4.
21. Leder SB, Ross DA. Confirmation of no causal relationship between tracheotomy and aspiration status: a direct replication study. Dysphagia. 2010;25:35–9.
22. Peterson SJ, Tsai AA, Scala CM. Adequacy of oral intake in critically ill patients 1 week after extubation. J Am Diet Assoc. 2010;110:427–33.
23. Skoretz SA, Flowers HL, Martino R. The incidence of dysphagia following endotracheal intubation. Chest. 2010;137:665–73.
24. Gordon C, Langton Hewer R, Wade DT. Dysphagia in acute stroke. BMJ. 1987;295:411–4.
25. Smithard DG, O'Neill PA, England RE, Park CL, Wyatt R, Martin DF, Morris J. The natural history of dysphagia following a stroke. Dysphagia. 1997;12:188–93.
26. McCullough GH, Wertz RT, Rosenbek JC, Dinnen C. Clinicians' prefernces and practices in conducting clinical/bedside and videofluoroscopic swallowing examinations in an adult, neurogenic population. Am J Speech Lang Pathol. 1999;8:149–63.
27. McCullough GH, Wertz RT, Rosenbek JC, Mills RH, Ross KB, Ashford JR. Inter- and intrajudge reliability of a clinical examination of swallowing in adults. Dysphagia. 2000;15:58–67.
28. Daniels SK. Optimal patterns of care for dysphagic stroke patients. Semin Speech Lang. 2000;21:323–31.
29. Leder SB, Suiter DM, Warner HL, Kaplan LJ. Initiating safe oral feeding in critically ill intensive care and step-down unit patients based on passing a 3-ounce (90 milliliters) water swallow challenge. J Trauma. 2011;70:1203–7.
30. DePippo KL, Holas MA, Reding MJ. The Burke dysphagia screening test: Validation of its use in patients with stroke. Arch Phys Med Rehabil. 1994;75:1284–6.

31. Chaves RD, de Carvalho RF, Cukier A, Stelmach R, de Andrade CRF. Symptoms of dysphagia in patients with COPD. J Bras Pneumol. 2011;37:76–83.
32. Martino R, Foley N, Bhogal S, Diamant N, Speechley M, Teasell R. Dysphagia after stroke: incidence, diagnosis, and pulmonary complications. Stroke. 2005;36:2756–63.
33. Barker J, Martino R, Reichardt B, Hickey EJ. Incidence and impact of dysphagia in patients receiving prolonged endotracheal intubation after cardiac surgery. Can J Surg. 2009;52:119–24.
34. Chouinard J. Dysphagia in Alzheimer disease: a review. J Nutr Health Aging. 2000;4:214–7.
35. Tjaden K. Speech and swallowing in Parkinson's disease. Top Geriatr Rehabil. 2008;24:115–26.
36. Leder SB, Novella S, Patwa H. Use of fiberoptic endoscopic evaluation of swallowing (FEES) in patients with amyotropohic lateral sclerosis. Dysphagia. 2004;19:177–81.
37. Tassorelli C, Bergamaschi R, Buscone S, Bartolo M, Furnari A, Crivelli P, Alfonsi E, Alberici E, Bertino G, Sandrini G, Nappi G. Dysphagia in multiple sclerosis: from pathogenesis to diagnosis. Neurol Sci. 2008;29 Suppl 4:S360–3.
38. Leder SB, Suiter DM, Warner HL, Acton LM, Swainson BA. Success of recommending oral diets in acute stroke patients based on a 90 cc water swallow challenge protocol. Top Stroke Rehabil. 2012;19:40–4.
39. Suiter DM, Leder SB, Karas DE. The 3-ounce (90 cc) water swallow challenge: a screening test for children with suspected oropharyngeal dysphagia. Otolaryngol Head Neck Surg. 2009;140:187–90.
40. Link DT, Willging JP, Miller CK. Pediatric laryngopharyngeal sensory testing during flexible endoscopic evaluation of swallowing: feasible and correlative. Ann Otol Rhinol Laryngol. 2000;109:899–905.
41. Donzelli J, Brady S, Wesling M. Predictive value of accumulated oropharyngeal secretions for aspiration during video nasal endoscopic evaluation of swallowing. Ann Otol Rhinol Laryngol. 2003;112:469–75.
42. Lazarus CL. Effects of chemoradiotherapy on voice and swallowing. Curr Opin Otolaryngol Head Neck Surg. 2009;17:172–8.

Chapter 7
Recommending Specific Oral Diets Based on Passing the Yale Swallow Protocol

Objectives: To discuss the rationale and implementation of recommending specific oral diets based on passing the Yale Swallow Protocol.

Methods: Synthesizing results of the 3-ounce water swallow challenge [1], the brief cognitive assessment [2], and oral mechanism examination [3] into a cohesive protocol.

Results: The Yale Swallow Protocol provides the clinician with a more nuanced and richer patient-oriented perspective on which to make timely and safe oral diet recommendations.

Conclusions: Important patient-specific factors need to be taken into account in order for an oral alimentation to be safe and successful. Once the protocol is passed ongoing mealtime monitoring is essential.

Keywords: Deglutition, Deglutition disorders, Swallow screening, Oral alimentation

Introduction

As important as determining aspiration risk is, recommending specific oral diets without the need for further instrumental dysphagia testing is an equally important goal of this programmatic

S.B. Leder and D.M. Suiter, *The Yale Swallow Protocol: An Evidence-Based Approach to Decision Making*, DOI 10.1007/978-3-319-05113-0_7, © Springer International Publishing Switzerland 2014

line of research. The Yale Swallow Protocol is the only screen with concomitant objective documentation from a large and heterogeneous population sample demonstrating a patient's swallowing ability with respect to food consistencies, i.e., thin liquid, puree, and solid (if dentate) consistency foods. As was shown in Suiter and Leder [1], the reason was that FEES was performed on all 3,000 patients immediately before the patient was required to perform the 3-ounce water swallow challenge component of the protocol. Therefore, it was known what specific food consistencies were swallowed successfully. This allows the clinician documentation on which to rely on to recommend and monitor a specific oral diet once the protocol was passed. For example, a thin liquid and puree diet if the patient has many missing teeth or is edentulous and a soft or regular consistency diet dependent upon the patient's cognitive abilities and dentition (natural or denture) status.

Synthesizing results of the 3-ounce water swallow challenge [1], the brief cognitive assessment [2], and oral mechanism examination [3] into a cohesive protocol provides the clinician with a more nuanced and richer patient-oriented perspective on which to make oral diet as well as compensatory feeding recommendations. As discussed in Chap. 6, the importance of clinical judgment and experience, in conjunction with information from the protocol, remains an essential factor in the care of the hospitalized and/or critically ill individual with suspected increased aspiration risk.

To briefly reiterate, important patient-specific factors need to be taken into account in order for an oral diet to be safe and successful. When possible, it is useful to know the patient's pre-morbid (pre-hospitalization) diet recommendations and feeding status, i.e., independent, assisted, or fed. This information can be obtained from the patient, family, or the extended care facility where the patient last lived. Once this is known an individualized patient care plan that is focused on the most appropriate diet can be fashioned. Therefore, successful application of protocol results entails both performing the screen correctly combined with appropriate interpretation of results in light of the patient's overall functioning.

Additionally, the clinician must be aware that patients of all ages who present with altered mental status, neurological impairment, traumatic brain injury, or stroke need to be evaluated and monitored regarding following directions, self-feeding skills, neglect, limb apraxia, nondominant upper extremity use, impulsivity, and task attentiveness. Many trauma patients become deconditioned and easily fatigued requiring diet modifications and assistance with oral intake. All patients, especially post-acute stroke and traumatic brain injury, are frustrated with new deficits and require in-depth assessment to determine specific diet modifications and rehabilitative needs for assistance with eating and feeding. Also, patients with swallowing problems uniformly benefit from encouragement and monitoring as work toward the goal of normal eating progresses. The dysphagia specialist, therefore, must synthesize objective, subjective, and behavioral data on an individual patient basis to promote safe and successful swallowing and eating.

Importance of Ongoing Monitoring

It must be remembered that a negative test allows for safe oral alimentation only as long as the patient remains medically and neurologically stable. Therefore, swallow screening or instrumental testing only provides a "snapshot in time" of a patient's swallowing abilities. Long-term swallowing success is never a guarantee [4]. For example, although infrequent, there may be times when after passing the protocol either the patient exhibits or nursing reports increased or inconsistent coughing during mealtimes and/or when taking medications in tablet form with liquids. This is not unexpected in both the acute care and rehabilitation settings. What is important is that the clinician uses any new information in order to make appropriate evidence-based recommendations for continued safe and successful oral alimentation.

When inconsistent but persistent coughing at mealtimes is observed the protocol should be readministered. This is one of the protocol's strengths as it is quick to administer, easy to interpret, and provides a definitive answer to aspiration risk status. If the protocol is passed again, oral alimentation can continue but the clinician should observe the patient at mealtimes and taking oral medications and, when appropriate, make recommendations that foster safer eating strategies, e.g., posture, rate of eating, bolus volume size, single swallows, and alternate liquid and solid consistency boluses.

Protocol failure indicates a potential change in the patient's medical or neurological status which may impact negatively on swallow function. The clinician should attempt to determine the etiology, e.g., altered mental status, fever, respiratory compromise, and fatigue, to determine if and when the protocol should be readministered. When the patient is at baseline or stable again, the clinician can choose to either readminister the protocol or proceed to further testing with FEES or VFSS. If the patient passes the protocol again, and armed with the knowledge of reports of inconsistent coughing at mealtimes, the clinician may recommend limiting thin liquid ingestion at mealtimes to single small, i.e., 5–10 cc, bolus volumes. It may also be the case that swallowing mixed consistencies at the same time is more problematic than swallowing one consistency at a time. Recommendations to ingest and swallow only one consistency at a time may eliminate prandial coughing. The goal, as always, is to reduce or eliminate potential aspiration risk. Chapter 11 focuses on additional information and discussion of longer-term monitoring of safe swallowing at mealtimes in the acute care setting.

Tablet Swallowing

Experienced dysphagia clinicians will recognize the unique difficulty of tablet swallowing. In fact, difficulty with tablet swallowing is not restricted to patients with dysphagia or deemed an aspiration risk as many people report difficulties. It is recommended that if the reports of inconsistent coughing are isolated to only when swallowing tablets, a discussion with the patient's physician regarding the possibility of changing medication formulation to liquid, crushable, or chewable is appropriate [5]. These changes often solve the problem.

References

1. Suiter DM, Leder SB. Clinical utility of the 3-ounce water swallow test. Dysphagia. 2008;23:244–50.
2. Leder SB, Suiter DM, Warner HL. Answering orientation questions and following single-step verbal commands: effect on aspiration status. Dysphagia. 2009;24:290–5.
3. Leder SB, Suiter DM, Murray J, Rademaker AW. Can an oral mechanism examination contribute to the assessment of odds of aspiration? Dysphagia. 2013;28:370–4.
4. Leder SB, Suiter DM, Warner HL, Kaplan LJ. Initiating safe oral feeding in critically ill intensive care and step-down unit patients based on passing a 3-ounce (90 milliliters) water swallow challenge. J Trauma. 2011;70:1203–7.
5. Leder SB, Lerner MZ. Nil per os except medications order in the dysphagic patient. Q J Med. 2013;106:71–5.

Chapter 8
Yale Swallow Protocol Administration and Interpretation: Passing and Failing

Objectives: To describe how to administer and interpret the Yale Swallow Protocol.

Methods: The development of three forms for the administration and interpretation of the protocol is provided. Step 1: Exclusion Criteria; Step 2: Administration and Instructions; and Step 3: Pass or Fail Criteria

Results: When to defer and when to administer the protocol as well as procedures to follow with either passing or failing the protocol are explained.

Conclusions: Three forms are provided for specific instructions for administration and interpretation of the Yale Swallow Protocol.

Keywords: Deglutition, Deglutition disorders, Swallow screening, Oral alimentation

Introduction

As with any other reliable and validated screening test used in medicine, once the Yale Swallow Protocol is passed the clinician should rely on its excellent operating characteristics and be confident that the patient is not an aspiration risk and, therefore, can begin oral alimentation and oral medications. The reader is referred to the detailed discussion on recommending oral diets in Chap. 7. Patients must be treated as unique individuals with specific strengths and weaknesses.

S.B. Leder and D.M. Suiter, *The Yale Swallow Protocol: An Evidence-Based* 105
Approach to Decision Making, DOI 10.1007/978-3-319-05113-0_8,
© Springer International Publishing Switzerland 2014

When all patient-specific factors are taken into consideration, e.g., diet, cognition and mental status, feeding ability, and posture, the clinician can formulate a plan to optimize successful eating.

Deferring Protocol Administration

Step 1 (Fig. 8.1) is a flow diagram used to determine if the protocol should be administered at all. The clinician should always read the patient's chart and talk with the primary treatment team. This is usually the RN or MD but ideally both. After adequate information is retrieved and if any one of the boxes is checked "No" protocol administration is deferred. The patient will then receive one of three recommendations: (1) An oral diet because no risk factors for aspiration are present; (2) An instrumental test because of a preexisting dysphagia or presence of a tracheotomy tube, or (3) Both protocol administration and instrumental testing are deferred because of head of bed restricted to <30°, inability to remain alert for testing, or nil-per-os order for medical/surgical reason.

Protocol Administration

We recommend that upon entering a patient's room for the first time the clinician establish good rapport by introducing themselves to the patient and any family or friend(s) that are present. After introductions, a statement as to the purpose of the protocol and what the patient will be required to do is explained.

Step 2 (Fig. 8.1) is comprised of the three components of the protocol. The patient is positioned upright at 90° or as upright as possible but >30° in a bed or chair and made comfortable.

First Component: The clinician performs a brief cognitive screen by asking the patient to state their name, where they are right now, and the current year. The clinician then asks the patient to open their mouth, stick out their tongue, and smile/pucker.

Second Component: The oral mechanism examination is performed where the patient is required to close their lips, move their tongue laterally from left to right labial commissure, and lastly smile and pucker.

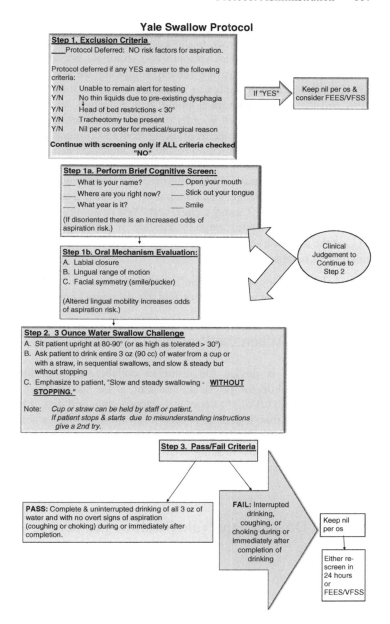

FIG. 8.1.   Yale Swallow Protocol flow diagram.

Third Component: Before beginning the 3-ounce challenge it is beneficial, but not mandatory, to dip a sponge swab into water in order to moisten the patient's mouth and stimulate one or two swallows. Then show the patient the cup containing the water and explain there is only 3 ounces in it and they have to drink it all, slow and steady, and without stopping. It is acceptable to repeat these instructions as needed in order to assure patient understanding. Give the patient a choice of drinking from the cup or using a straw as neither delivery method resulted in increased aspiration of water [1]. Either hand them the cup to drink or assist them with holding the cup or straw while drinking. Use verbal encouragement during the challenge, i.e., "Suck it up" (if using a straw), or "Keep on drinking" (if using a cup), and "You're doing great" to ensure uninterrupted and complete drinking. It is also acceptable to give the patient a second chance at drinking the 3 ounces based upon clinician discretion.

Step 3 (Fig. 8.1) includes the results and interpretation template. Directions to follow with a Pass or Fail are delineated below.

What to Do When the Protocol Is Passed

If the protocol is passed the clinician collaborates with the patient's medical doctor, physician assistant, or licensed independent provider (MD/PA/LIP) to order the appropriate oral diet. It is usually the case that, if dentate or only a few missing teeth, a soft solid consistency or regular consistency diet can be ordered and, if edentulous or many missing teeth, a liquid and puree diet. Chapter 7 provides a detailed discussion on recommending specific oral diets based on passing the Yale Swallow Protocol.

What to Do When the Yale Swallow Protocol Is Failed

The clinician has two options if the Yale Swallow Protocol is failed. Option 1 is to keep the patient nil per os (including medications) and inform the MD/PA/LIP that an instrumental swallowing evaluation is required. There are two instrumental testing choices. First, a FEES examination can be done by speech-language pathology immediately at the bedside. Second, later that day a VFSS can be done by speech-language pathology and diagnostic radiology in the fluoroscopy suite. This will permit diagnosing dysphagia and for appropriate recommendations to be made regarding either continued nil-per-os status or initiating oral feeding trials. There is evidence for good success for oral alimentation with some form of a modified diet or feeding regimen as 71 % of patients who fail the challenge are nevertheless able to tolerate a modified volume and/or modified consistency diet [2, 3].

Option 2 is to recommend continued nil-per-os status (with or without IV hydration and/or tube feedings dependent upon medical condition) and repeat the protocol in 24 h. Many acute care hospitalized patients make rapid progress in 24 h and repeat testing, when medically and neurologically appropriate, has been shown to be beneficial in implementing timely, safe, and successful oral alimentation [4]. If subsequently passed, it is appropriate to recommend an oral diet as per protocol interpretation. If failed again, however, a discussion regarding treatment options with the patient's physician should occur; specifically, the need to continue nil-per-os status for a third protocol administration in another 24 h, when to start enteral tube feedings, or when to perform an instrumental test (FEES or VFSS) dependent upon the patient's medical and neurological condition, goals of care, cognitive status, and likelihood of both safety and success with oral alimentation trials.

References

1. Veiga HP, Fonseca HV, Bianchini EMG. Sequential swallowing of liquid in elderly adults: cup or straw? Dysphagia. 2014;29:249–55.
2. Suiter DM, Leder SB. Clinical utility of the 3-ounce water swallow test. Dysphagia. 2008;23:244–50.
3. Leder SB, Judson BL, Sliwinski E, Madson L. Promoting safe swallowing when puree is swallowed without aspiration but thin liquid is aspirated: nectar is enough. Dysphagia. 2013;28:58–62.
4. Leder SB. Serial fiberoptic endoscopic swallowing evaluations in the management of patients with dysphagia. Arch Phys Med Rehabil. 1998;79:1264–9.

Chapter 9
Implementation of the Yale Swallow Protocol by Other Health-Care Professionals

One of the key goals of any screening instrument is simplicity of administration and interpretation by screeners with varying amounts of expertise. After all, its use will be severely limited if only highly trained personnel are able to use it. It is very important, therefore, to determine if other health-care providers, besides speech-language pathologists, can both administer and interpret the Yale Swallow Protocol efficiently, reliably, and correctly. Only then will the protocol have gained stature as a screening tool that not only has adequate validity and reliability but also widespread generalizability and utility in regard to both patients and clinicians.

Warner HL, Suiter DM, Nystrom K, Poskus K, Leder SB. Comparing accuracy of the 3-ounce water swallow challenge dysphagia screening protocol when administered by registered nurses and speech-language pathologists. Journal of Clinical Nursing doi: 10.1111/jocn.12340 (In Press). (Used and modified with permission from John Wiley & Sons Ltd.)

Objectives: Avoidance of potentially preventable prandial pulmonary aspiration as a cause of nosocomial infection is an important goal for all acute care hospitalized patients deemed at risk for aspiration. However, current nurse administered swallow screens use a variety of nonevidence-based assessments making early identification of potential swallowing problems problematic. The purpose of the present study was to determine the accuracy of the Yale Swallow Protocol comprised of a brief cognitive screen [1], an oral mechanism evaluation [2], and drinking 3 ounces of water [3],

S.B. Leder and D.M. Suiter, *The Yale Swallow Protocol: An Evidence-Based*   111
Approach to Decision Making, DOI 10.1007/978-3-319-05113-0_9,
© Springer International Publishing Switzerland 2014

when administered and interpreted by registered nurses and compared with blinded ratings from speech-language pathology.

Methods: Two speech-language pathologists, 52 registered nurses, and 101 inpatients participated. First, each participant was administered the Yale Swallow Protocol by a speech-language pathologist. Second, a nurse administered the protocol to the same patient within 1 h and independently recorded results and diet recommendations. The nurse was blinded to the study's purpose and results of the speech-language pathologist's initial screening. Out of view, but simultaneous with the nurse administered protocol, another speech-language pathologist re-rated the patient's challenge for comparison with initial results and determined accuracy of the nurse administered protocol.

Results: Intra- and inter-rater protocol agreements for the two speech-language pathologists were 100 %. Inter-rater protocol agreement between registered nurses and speech-language pathologists was 98.01 % with a Cohen's Kappa of 0.95. Results confirmed the reliability and accuracy of a registered nurse administered and interpreted swallow screening protocol.

Conclusions: The consequence of 98 % registered nurse accuracy combined with previously reported 96.5 % sensitivity, 97.9 % negative predictive value, and <2 % false negative rate allowed for adoption of the Yale Swallow Protocol for the entire general hospital population.

Keywords: Deglutition, Deglutition disorders, Aspiration, Acute care, Multi-professional care, Screening tool, Oral alimentation

Introduction

Reliable swallowing screening for potential aspiration risk requires use of a validated and reliable test administered by trained personnel. As stated previously in Chap. 2, a successful swallow screen should be simple to administer, cross-disciplinary, cost effective, acceptable to patients, and able to identify the target attribute by giving a positive finding when aspiration risk is present and a negative finding when dysphagia is absent [4]. Following these established guidelines, only a reliable, repeatable, evidence-based, and cost-effective screening test with acceptable risk assessment values for determination of the presence of aspiration risk should be used [5, 6].

Avoidance of potentially preventable adverse events, such as prandial aspiration pneumonia, is a priority in hospitalized patients making early identification of potential swallowing prob-lems leading to aspiration risk an important goal prior to oral ingestion of food, fluids, and medications. The need for recognition of swallowing difficulties early in a patient's hospital stay supports the need for an evidence-based, registered nurse (RN) administered swallow screen [7]. RNs have an opportunity to change outcomes positively as they are often the first health-care professionals to assess and care for patients admitted into an acute health-care environment. Since a gastrointestinal assessment, which includes ability to take oral nutrition, is already a component of the nursing admission assessment for all hospitalized patients, it seems only reasonable to have an easily administered, validated, and reliable swallow screen that can be administered by trained RNs to the majority of hospitalized patients.

RNs already screen patients for swallowing problems and aspiration risk [8] but, unfortunately, with a variety of nonevidence-based assessment tools. Screens have included a questionnaire followed by three teaspoons and a glass of water [9, 10], a neuro-logical assessment followed by teaspoons of lemon ice, apple sauce, and water [11], a questionnaire then a 90 cc water swallow but only if no dysphagia indicators are present [12], and a decision tree incorporating applesauce, increasing sips of water, and a cracker [13]. However, the accuracy of these clinical screens, specifically their ability to identify the target attribute by giving a positive finding when aspiration risk is present and a negative finding when aspiration risk is absent [4], is unknown because no instrumental reference standard, i.e., FEES or VFSS, was used to corroborate accuracy and determine acceptable sensitivity scores, negative predictive values, and false negative rates [5, 6].

If RNs were able to reliably administer and interpret The Yale Swallow Protocol, timely initiation of specific diet recommendations

TABLE 9.1.   Patient demographics ($n = 101$) (used with permission from John Wiley & Sons Ltd: Warner HL, Suiter DM, Nystrom K, Poskus, K, Leder SB).

Age (year)	Gender	Diagnosis	n
$\bar{X} = 62.45$	54M/47F	Cardiothoracic surgery	6
SD = 17.41		Medical	18
Range: 18–94		Pulmonary	15
		Cancer	3
		Non-neurologic $n=$	42
		Left stroke	10
		Right stroke	8
		Neurosurgery	10
		Other neurologic[a]	31
		Neurologic $n=$	59
		Total $n=$	101

Comparing accuracy of the 3-ounce water swallow challenge dysphagia screening protocol when administered by registered nurses and speech-language pathologists. J Clin Nurs doi: 10.1111/jocn.12340 In Press: 2014

[a]Traumatic brain injury, brain tumor, epilepsy, seizure disorder, degenerative

and oral medications could be made in virtually all hospitalized patients. The purpose of the present study was to determine the accuracy of the RN administered Yale Swallow Protocol when compared with concurrent ratings from speech-language pathology.

Two speech-language pathologists, 52 RNs, and 101 inpatients from a large, urban, acute care, teaching hospital participated. In order to reduce selection bias, RN participation was not based on experience or degree status beyond RN. Inclusion criteria for all RNs were assignment to care of the patient participant. Table 9.1 shows patient demographics including age, gender, and admitting diagnosis. The standard protocol administration and inclusion and exclusion criteria as in Leder et al. [14–16] were used.

Within 1 h of the initial protocol administration by the speech-language pathologist, an RN administered the 3-ounce water challenge to the same patient and independently recorded results and diet recommendations. The RN was blinded to both the purpose of the study and to the results of the speech-language pathologist's initial 3-ounce challenge. Out of view but simultaneous with the RN administered water swallow challenge, another speech-language

TABLE 9.2.   Intra- and inter-rater agreements for speech-language pathology and RNs.

Intra-rater agreement	
Speech-language pathologist # 1 (based on 26 screens)	100 %
Speech-language pathologist # 2 (based on 75 screens)	100 %
Inter-rater agreement	
Speech-language pathologists # 1 and # 2 v. RNs (based on 101 screens)	98.01 %

Used with permission from John Wiley & Sons Ltd: Warner HL, Suiter DM, Nystrom K, Poskus, K, Leder SB. Comparing accuracy of the 3-ounce water swallow challenge dysphagia screening protocol when administered by registered nurses and speech-language pathologists. J Clin Nurs doi: 10.1111/jocn.12340 In Press: 2014

pathologist both re-rated the patient's 3-ounce water swallow challenge for comparison with their initial results and determined the accuracy of the RN administered challenge protocol, scoring, and diet recommendations.

Table 9.2 shows intra- and inter-rater agreements. Intra-rater agreement for the two speech-language pathologists was determined by comparing their respective initial 3-ounce challenge protocol results (one speech-language pathologist performed 26 screens and the other speech-language pathologist performed 75 screens) with results of the observed challenge protocol administered by the RNs. Inter-rater agreement between the two speech-language pathologists and RNs was determined by comparing results of the observed challenge with results of the RNs administration and independent ratings of the challenge ($n = 101$). Both intra- and inter-rater agreements for the two speech-language pathologists were 100 %. Inter-rater agreement between the RNs and speech-language pathologists was 98.01 %. Additionally, Cohen's kappa was determined to be 1.0 for intra- and inter-rater SLP agreement and 0.95 for inter-rater RN and SLP agreement. These values are judged to be excellent agreement.

Table 9.3 shows RN pass/fail ratings by participant diagnosis. The same RN (who was later retrained) passed two participants incorrectly when interrupted drinking occurred, i.e., one with a diagnosis of left stroke and one with a diagnosis of other neurologic (seizure disorder). No diagnostic category was associated with increased difficulty during administration and interpretation of the 3-ounce water swallow challenge protocol.

TABLE 9.3. RN pass/fail results of the 3-ounce water swallow challenge protocol dependent upon diagnosis ($n = 101$).

Diagnosis	n	Pass	Fail
Cardiothoracic surgery	6	4	2
Medical	18	16	2
Pulmonary	15	10	5
Cancer	3	2	1
Left stroke	10	4[a]	6
Right stroke	8	4	4
Neurosurgery	10	8	2
Other neurologic[b]	31	24[a]	7
Total	101	72	29

Used with permission from John Wiley & Sons Ltd: Warner HL, Suiter DM, Nystrom K, Poskus, K, Leder SB. Comparing accuracy of the 3-ounce water swallow challenge dysphagia screening protocol when administered by registered nurses and speech-language pathologists. J Clin Nurs doi: 10.1111/jocn.12340 In Press: 2014
[a]RN incorrectly passed patient when interrupted drinking occurred
[b]Traumatic brain injury, brain tumor, degenerative, epilepsy, seizure disorder

This is the first report of use of a highly accurate RN administered swallow screen based on a previously validated, evidence-based, and cost-effective protocol with acceptable risk assessment values for determination of potential aspiration risk. The consequence of 98 % RN accuracy combined with 96.5 % sensitivity, 97.9 % negative predictive value [3], and a <2 % false negative rate [17] is that the Yale Swallow Protocol has been adopted as standard practice not only on the neurological service [15] but for the entire general hospital population [16]. The electronic medical record was, therefore, revised to allow RNs to document results of the swallow screening protocol at several points in the admitting process, i.e., in the emergency department, upon arrival in the unit, and at any time a change in medical status was observed. An adverse preventable event such as prandial aspiration pneumonia can be potentially avoided due to the ability to monitor oral intake status at any point during the patient's hospitalization.

Conclusions

In conclusion, the result of this study [18] confirmed both the reliability and accuracy of the Yale Swallow Protocol when administered and interpreted by an RN and adds to the evidence supporting its adoption as standard practice for the entire general hospital population [16]. Correct use of this protocol by RNs allows for early identification of potential swallowing problems. Passing results in timely ingestion of food, liquid, and medication. Failing results in nil-per-os status and triggers a referral to speech-language pathology for further evaluation.

References

1. Suiter DB, Leder SB. Clinical utility of the 3 ounce water swallow test. Dysphagia. 2008;23:244–50.
2. Leder SB, Suiter DM, Murray J, Rademaker AW. Can an oral mechanism examination contribute to the assessment of odds of aspiration? Dysphagia. 2013;28:370–3.
3. Leder SB, Suiter DM, Warner HL. Answering orientation questions and following single step verbal commands: effect on aspiration status. Dysphagia. 2009;24:290–5.
4. Cochrane AL, Holland WW. Validation of screening procedures. British Med Bull. 1971;27:3–8.
5. McCullough GH, Wertz RT, Rosenbek JC, Dinneen C. Clinicians' Preferences and practices in conducting clinical/bedside and videofluoroscopic swallowing examinations in adult, neurogenic population. Am J Speech Lang Pathol. 1999;8:149–63.
6. McCullough GH, Wertz RT, Rosenbek JC, Mills RH, Ross KB, Ashford JR. Inter-and intrajudge reliability of a clinical examination of swallowing in adults. Dysphagia. 2000;15:58–67.
7. Bours GJJ, Speyer R, Lemmens J, Limburg M, de Wit R. Bedside screening tests vs. Videofluoroscopy or fiberoptic endoscopic evaluation of swallowing to detect dysphagia in patients with neurological disorders: systematic review. J Adv Nurs. 2008;65:477–93.
8. Hines S, Wallace K, Crowe L, Finlayson K, Chang A, Pattie M. Identification and nursing management of dysphagia in individuals with acute neurological impairment (update). Int J Evid Based Healthc. 2011;9:148–50.
9. Perry L. Screening swallowing function of patients with acute stroke. Part one: identification, implementation and initial evaluation of a screening tool for use by nurses. J Clin Nurs. 2001;10:463–73.

10. Perry L. Screening swallowing function of patients with acute stroke. Part two: detailed evaluation of the tool used by nurses. J Clin Nurs. 2001;10:474–81.

11. Weinhardt J, Hazelett S, Barrett D, Lada R, Enos T, Keleman R. Accuracy of a bedside dysyphagia screening: a comparison of registered nurses and speech therapists. Rehabil Nurs. 2008;33:247–52.

12. Cichero JAY, Heaton S, Bassett L. Triaging dysphagia: nurse screening for dysphagia in an acute hospital. J Clin Nurs. 2009;18:1649–59.

13. Barnard SL, Hohenhaus SM. Nursing dysphagia screening for acute stroke patients in the emergency department. J Emerg Nurs. 2011; 37:64–7.

14. Leder SB, Suiter DM, Warner HL, Kaplan LJ. Initiating safe oral feeding in critically ill intensive care and step-down unit patients based on passing a 3-ounce (90 milliliters) water swallow challenge. J Trauma. 2011;70:1203–7.

15. Leder SB, Suiter DM, Warner HL, Acton LM, Siegel MD. Safe initiation of oral diets in hospitalized patients based on passing a 3-ounce (90 cc) water swallow challenge protocol. Q J Med. 2012;105:257–63.

16. Leder SB, Suiter DM, Warner HL, Acton LM, Swainson BA. Success of recommending oral diets in acute stroke patients based on a 90-cc water swallow challenge protocol. Top Stroke Rehabil. 2012;19:40–4.

17. Leder SB, Suiter DM, Green BG. Silent aspiration risk is volume dependent. Dysphagia. 2011;26:304–9.

18. Warner HL, Suiter DM, Nystrom K, Poskus, K, Leder SB. Comparing accuracy of the 3-ounce water swallow challenge dysphagia screening protocol when administered by registered nurses and speech-language pathologists. J Clin Nur. doi: 10.1111/jocn.12340 (in press): 2014.

Chapter 10
Question: What About Silent Aspiration? Answer: Silent Aspiration Is Volume-Dependent

A swallow screen's most important objective is determination of the probability of aspiration risk. This is done by examination of the screen's statistical operating characteristics as discussed in Chap. 2. It is not to diagnose dysphagia which is the purview of instrumental FEES and VFSS testing. It cannot be stressed enough that a screen cannot determine pharyngeal and laryngeal anatomy and physiology or bolus flow characteristics. This is why a high sensitivity, a high negative predictive value, and a low false negative rate for the determination of aspiration risk are so crucial to the reliability of a swallow screen. An important aspect of any swallow screen, therefore, must be able to mitigate the probability of missing silent aspiration.

Silent aspiration is defined as when food or fluids enter the airway and travel below the level of the true vocal folds without eliciting a protective cough response in an attempt to expel the material [1]. Therefore, if silent aspiration occurs it is undetectable, by definition, during a bedside assessment because there are no overt signs to indicate its occurrence. However, silent aspiration is important because unrecognized prandial aspiration has the potential to result in pneumonia which can increase the incidences of both morbidity and mortality.

S.B. Leder and D.M. Suiter, *The Yale Swallow Protocol: An Evidence-Based*   119
Approach to Decision Making, DOI 10.1007/978-3-319-05113-0_10,
© Springer International Publishing Switzerland 2014

Here are the facts about what a swallow screen is unable to determine:

1. *No swallow screen can identify when or even if silent aspiration has occurred.* The reason is the patient does not give any overt behavioral signs that an aspiration event has occurred.
2. *No swallow screen can provide information on pharyngeal and laryngeal anatomy or physiology.* The reason is it is impossible to view the pharynx and larynx without instrumentation. And it is inappropriate to infer physiological functioning from acoustic information. Strictly speaking, there is no 1:1 correspondence between individual motor acts and specific acoustic events [2]. For example, a breathy vocal quality may be indicative of unilateral true vocal fold impairment, bilateral true vocal fold impairment, mass effect on one or both true vocal folds, or true vocal fold bowing, all of which contribute to the acoustic signature of a breathy vocal quality.
3. *No swallow screen can determine bolus flow characteristics.* The reason is that without visualization bolus flow rate to determine pre-swallow spillage or delayed triggering of the pharyngeal swallow cannot be determined. Therefore, pre-swallow pooling or post-swallow residue in the valleculae, pyriform sinuses, and laryngeal vestibule is unknowable.

As a result, it behooves the clinician to use a swallow screen that eliminates as much as possible the potential to miss silent aspiration. Screens that use non-swallowing tasks such as questionnaires or behavioral signs not associated with swallowing like facial droop, gag reflex, or dysarthria cannot do this. Screens that use swallowing tasks that do not stress the limits of the swallowing system by using small 5 or 10 cc (or less!) bolus volumes cannot do this. Therefore, a screen must use a swallowing task of sufficient difficulty so as to stress the swallow system to such an extent that the risk of silent aspiration occurring is reduced to the low single digit percentages. The Yale Swallow Protocol is just such a screen and is supported by evidence-based research.

Leder SB, Suiter DM, Green BG. Silent aspiration risk is volume dependent. Dysphagia. 2011;26:304–9. (Used and modified with kind permission from Springer Science + Business Media.)

Objectives: Clinical swallow protocols cannot detect silent aspiration due to absence of overt behavioral signs, but screening with a much larger bolus volume, i.e., 90 cc vs. 1–10 cc, may elicit a reflexive cough in individuals who might otherwise exhibit silent aspiration. A swallow screen that maintains high sensitivity to identify aspiration risk while simultaneously reducing the false negative rate for silent aspiration would be beneficial to patient care. The purpose of this study was to investigate whether silent aspiration risk was volume-dependent by using a 3-ounce water swallow challenge to elicit a reflexive cough when silent aspiration occurred on much smaller bolus volumes.

Methods: A prospective, consecutive, referral-based sample of 4,102 inpatients from the acute care setting of a large urban tertiary care teaching participated. Silent aspiration was determined first by FEES and then each participant was instructed to drink 3 ounces of water completely and without interruption. Criteria for challenge failure were inability to drink the entire amount, stopping and starting, or coughing and choking during or immediately after completion.

Results: Improved identification of aspiration risk status occurred for 58 % of participants who exhibited silent aspiration on smaller volumes, i.e., an additional 48 % of liquid silent aspirators and 65.6 % of puree silent aspirators coughed when attempting the 3-ounce water swallow challenge. A low overall false negative rate was observed for the entire population sample, i.e., ≤ 2.0 %. A combined false negative rate for participants who silently aspirated was 6.9 %, i.e., 7.8 % if silently aspirated liquid and 6.1 % if silently aspirated puree consistency. In-depth analysis of individual participant data indicated that the majority of silent aspiration was categorized as trace amounts and such small volumes do not influence diet recommendations or feeding strategies.

Conclusions: Determination of silent aspiration risk was shown to be volume-dependent with a larger volume eliciting a reflexive cough in individuals who previously silently aspirated on smaller volumes. A 3-ounce water swallow challenge's previously reported high sensitivity for identification of aspiration risk combined with the newly reported low false negative rate mitigates the issue of silent aspiration risk during clinical swallow screening.

Keywords: Deglutition, Deglutition disorders, Aspiration risk, Swallow screening, Oral alimentation

Introduction

Comparing studies dealing with silent aspiration is problematic due to differences in methodology and population samples and, most importantly, varying stimuli used to detect silent aspiration. Despite these challenges, instrumental confirmation of silent aspiration occurs frequently: 15–39 % in individuals following stroke [3–5]; 25–52 % in adults referred for swallowing evaluations in the acute primary care setting [1, 6, 7]; 77–82 % in individuals who require mechanical ventilation [8, 9]; and 94 % in children with developmental disabilities [10].

The clinical swallow screen cannot detect silent aspiration because, by definition and as discussed above, visual confirmation is required in the absence of overt behavioral signs [11, 12]. It may be possible, however, to mitigate this requirement. The literature shows that only small bolus volumes, ranging from 1 to 10 cc, have been used when investigating silent aspiration during objective testing with either VFSS or FEES [1, 6–10, 13–16]. Only three studies have mentioned a volume effect relative to aspiration, with silent aspiration invariably associated with trace amounts of aspirate, defined as less than 10 % of (an already small) bolus volume [10, 17, 18]. This small amount of aspirate does not preclude oral alimentation [18]. It has been conjectured that aspiration of such small volumes may not provide an adequate stimulus to trigger a cough reflex in healthy older adults [17] as well as in many patient populations, e.g., patients with dementia, neurological sequelae, receiving sedating medications, following surgery and chemo-radiation therapy for head and neck cancer, or after long-term endotracheal intubation and tracheotomy.

Research on irritant receptors has shown that water has the capacity to stimulate laryngeal and tracheal receptors in several different ways: via mechanical stimulation [19–22]; via temperature changes, i.e., cooling [23, 24]; due to hypo-osmolality [25]; and following removal of chloride ions [26]. Increasing the bolus

TABLE 10.1.   Participant demographics (used with kind permission from Springer Science + Business Media: Leder SB, Suiter DM, Green BG. Silent aspiration risk is volume dependent. Dysphagia. 26:304–9, 2011).

Gender[a]	
Females	$N = 1,780$ (43.5 %)
Males	$N = 2,314$ (56.5 %)
Age[b]	
Females	$\bar{X} = 70.30$ years (range = 2.0–105.0 years)
Males	$\bar{X} = 66.27$ years (range = 2.2–105.0 years)

[a]Data are missing for 8 (0.2 %) participants
[b]Data are missing for 20 (0.5 %) participants

volume used in a swallowing challenge has the potential to increase each of these forms of stimulation by providing a larger volume of water to be aspirated.

Therefore, a swallow challenge utilizing a much larger bolus volume, i.e., 90 cc (3 oz.) vs. 1–10 cc, may increase sensitivity by triggering an aspiration-related cough reflex in individuals who might otherwise exhibit silent aspiration. The false negative rate, i.e., the proportion of disease (in this case aspiration) missed by the test, would be reduced, thereby mitigating the issue of silent aspiration risk during the clinical swallow screen.

A swallow screen that maintains high sensitivity to identify aspiration risk [27] while simultaneously reducing the false negative rate for silent aspiration risk would be beneficial. The purpose of the present study was to investigate whether silent aspiration risk is volume-dependent by using a 3-ounce water swallow challenge [27] to enhance identification of aspiration risk status by triggering the cough reflex in those individuals who exhibit silent aspiration on smaller bolus volumes.

A prospective, consecutive, referral-based sample of 4,102 inpatients from the acute care setting of a large urban tertiary care teaching hospital were evaluated objectively with FEES. All participants were given the 3-ounce water swallow challenge. However, due to severe dysphagia and documented aspiration 313 participants were deemed unsafe to be given thin liquids and 110 deemed unsafe to be given puree consistency during FEES. Table 10.1 shows participant demographics and Table 10.2 shows admitting diagnostic categories.

TABLE 10.2.   Diagnostic categories   (used with kind permission from Springer Science + Business Media: Leder SB, Suiter DM, Green BG. Silent aspiration risk is volume dependent. Dysphagia. 26:304–9, 2011).

Diagnostic category[a]	Number
Cancer	168
Cardiothoracic surgery	220
Dementia	127
Esophageal surgery	78
Head and neck surgery	172
Medical	1,214
Neurological (traumatic brain injury/other)	497
Neurosurgery	317
Parkinson's disease	30
Pulmonary	642
Stroke (left hemisphere)	302
Stroke (right hemisphere)	262
Stroke (brainstem)	54

[a]Data are missing for 19 (0.5 %) participants

The standard FEES protocol as in Suiter and Leder [27] was followed. A 100 % non-blinded agreement between the endoscopist (SBL) and assisting health-care professional, e.g., physician, physician assistant, speech-language pathologist, registered nurse, or respiratory therapist, was required to confirm silent aspiration status.

Immediately following completion of FEES, the endoscopist administered a 3-ounce water swallow challenge [27]. Each participant was given 3 ounces of water and instructed to drink the entire amount, via cup or straw, completely and without interruption. A 100 % non-blinded agreement between the endoscopist and assisting health-care professional was required to confirm results of the water swallow, i.e., criteria for challenge failure included inability to drink the entire amount, stopping and starting, or coughing and choking during or immediately after completion.

Confirmatory intra- and inter-rater reliability testing was performed prospectively with 128 additional cases. Two speech-language pathologists experienced in interpreting FEES results independently and blindly reviewed the swallows on a digital swallowing workstation (Kay Elemetrics Corp., Model 7200). Using real-time analysis with repeat viewing as needed, both

TABLE 10.3.   Volume-dependent aspiration risk (used with kind permission from Springer Science+Business Media: Leder SB, Suiter DM, Green BG. Silent aspiration risk is volume dependent. Dysphagia. 26:304–9, 2011).

FEES results

Liquid aspiration=761/3,789[a] (20.1 %)	Puree aspiration=559/3,992[b] (14.0 %)
Cough=595/761 (78.2 %)	Cough=379/560 (67.9 %)
Silent=166/761 (21.8 %)	Silent=180/560 (32.1 %)
Combined silent aspirators=346/1,321 (26.2 %)	

3-ounce water challenge results

Could not complete=132/166 (79.5 %)	Could not complete=143/180 (79.4 %)
Passed=13/25[c] (52 %)	Passed=11/32[d] (34.4 %)
Cough=12/25 (48 %)	Cough=21/32 (65.6 %)
Combined volume effect=33/57 (58.0 %)	

False negative results

3-ounce challenge vs. liquid aspiration	3-ounce challenge vs. puree aspiration
Passed vs. total (13/761=1.7 %)	Passed vs. total (11/560=2.0 %)
Passed vs. silent (13/166=7.8 %)	Passed vs. silent (11/180=6.1 %)
Combined silent false negatives=24/346 (6.9 %)	

[a] It was deemed unsafe to give 313 participants thin liquid consistency boluses based on FEES results but they all participated in the 3-ounce water swallow challenge

[b] It was deemed unsafe to give 110 participants puree consistency boluses based on FEES results but they all participated in the 3-ounce water swallow challenge

[c] 9/34 (26.5 %) participants exhibited trace aspiration on FEES and were excluded

[d] 5/37 (13.5 %) participants exhibited trace aspiration on FEES and were excluded

intra- and inter-rater reliability ratings for tracheal aspiration were 100 %. Subsequent randomized and double-blinded determination of aspiration status using the 3-ounce challenge and VFSS confirmed the 100 % identification of tracheal aspiration [28].

Table 10.3 shows volume-dependent aspiration risk results. Accurate identification of aspiration risk was enhanced for 33 of 57 (58 %) participants who previously exhibited silent aspiration on smaller volumes. Specifically, an additional 12 of 25 (48 %) liquid silent aspirators and 21 of 32 (65.6 %) puree silent aspirators coughed when attempting the 3-ounce water swallow challenge.

A low false negative rate of ≤2.0 % was observed for the entire population sample, i.e., participants who passed a 3-ounce challenge but aspirated liquid or puree consistency on FEES. A combined false negative rate for participants who silently aspirated was 6.9 %, i.e., 7.8 % if silently aspirated liquid consistency and 6.1 % if silently aspirated puree consistency.

Volume-dependent determination of aspiration risk status occurred and a volume effect relative to identification of silent aspiration risk established. Specifically, an additional 58 % of participants who exhibited silent aspiration on small ($\leq$5 cc) liquid and puree bolus volumes during FEES exhibited overt aspiration risk behavior, i.e., cough, when required to drink 3 ounces of water in sequential swallows without stopping. Elicitation of the cough reflex in individuals who previously exhibited silent aspiration on smaller bolus volumes enhanced the clinical identification of aspiration risk status.

It has been shown that sequential cup [18] and straw [29] drinking increases upper airway penetration and, therefore, aspiration risk. Specifically, both laryngeal penetration and tracheal aspiration scores were significantly higher with sequential vs. single swallows [30] and increased aspiration risk due to laryngeal penetration was exhibited in 59 % of a cohort of non-dysphagic subjects ranging in age from 21 to 103 years [18]. It was reported that patients who exhibited aspiration with small single bolus volumes were at even higher aspiration risk during larger sequential drinking [30]. Consequently, participants classified as false negatives, i.e., aspiration on FEES but no cough with a 3-ounce challenge (Table 10.3), were considered to be at increased aspiration risk [18, 29, 31, 32].

The overall mean silent aspiration rate of 26.2 % with FEES (Table 10.3) was consistent with the literature when small bolus volumes ($\leq$10 cc) were used in testing, i.e., 25–52 % of adults referred for swallowing evaluations in the acute primary care setting exhibited silent aspiration [1, 6, 7]. Also consistent with previous results, over 75 % of participants who exhibited silent aspiration could not complete a 3-ounce challenge due to generalized deconditioning, dementia, or neurological sequelae [27]. Lastly, silent aspiration occurred over 10 % more often with puree consistency (32.1 %) vs. liquid (21.8 %) consistency.

As noted earlier, larger water bolus volumes should, in principle, increase the probability of evoking a cough reflex due to aspiration via a number of different sensory mechanisms. Although some laryngeal mechanoreceptors are exquisitely sensitive to punctate mechanical stimulation [33], neurological damage in clinical populations may effectively decrease the afferent signal, necessitating stronger and/or more spatially extensive stimulation to exceed the sensory threshold of the cough reflex. A larger volume of water would be capable of producing a stronger afferent discharge both by virtue of its greater mass (and thus stronger mechanical pressure) and via spatial summation. Spatial summation, in which sensation increases in proportion to the total area of stimulation, has been demonstrated to be ample in cutaneous mechanoreception [34–36], though it has not yet been studied in visceral mechanoreception. Similarly, spatial summation is a significant factor in cutaneous cold sensitivity [37, 38], and the greater heat capacity of larger volumes of water would, by itself, deliver a more potent cooling stimulus to laryngeal cold receptors [24]. Finally, larger water volumes increase the likelihood that aspiration would reduce the osmolality [25] and chloride concentration [26] of the airway mucosa sufficiently to stimulate laryngeal receptors. The latter changes would also be expected to take place over larger areas of mucosa, effectively producing a spatial summation of these factors as well.

There were a small number of false negatives (≤ 2 %), which is as expected when screening a large and heterogeneous population sample. Detailed inspection of these participants revealed that one-quarter to one-third of the false negative aspiration events were categorized as *trace* amounts, i.e., when less than an estimated 10 % of the (already small ≤ 5 cc) bolus volume was observed below the level of the true vocal folds [10, 17]. For research purposes, the presence of trace aspiration mandated categorizing a participant as exhibiting aspiration on FEES. From a clinical perspective, however, these patients would not be considered false negatives as this very small amount of aspirate did not automatically trigger discontinuance of the evaluation [18] or preclude recommending oral alimentation. Proceeding with testing allowed for the determination of continued aspiration and if aspiration was consistency specific, e.g., only occurred on thin liquids. In no case was nil-per-os status recommended when only trace aspiration was observed [10] as all participants who exhibited trace aspiration were recommended for and successful with an oral diet [18, 38]. Therefore, in reality the already low ≤ 2 % false negative rate is, in all likelihood, actually lower.

Patients who require a tracheotomy tube for respiration and pulmonary toilet should not be tested with a 3-ounce water swallow challenge. Silent aspiration occurs more frequently due to laryngeal desensitization from chronic aspiration of secretions [39, 40], the effects of chemo-radiation therapy [41], and, although a tracheotomy is not causal for aspiration [42, 43] if aspiration occurs it is often silent, leading to higher false negative rates. Therefore, instrumental testing with VFSS or FEES is recommended for these patients.

Conclusions

In conclusion, use of 3 ounces of water as a component in a protocol with the purpose of screening for aspiration risk has been strengthened. Use of a direct swallowing task and of sufficient volume is a requisite. For the first time, determination of silent aspiration risk was shown to be volume-dependent with a larger volume eliciting a reflexive cough in individuals who previously aspirated silently on smaller volumes. The protocol's strength to reduce the false negative rate for silent aspiration risk to very low single digit levels combined with its previously documented high sensitivity (96.5 %) and negative predictive values (97.9 %) to identify aspiration risk [27] makes it a highly effective and extremely sensitive screening tool. Correct use of the Yale Swallow Protocol mitigates the issue of silent aspiration risk during clinical swallow screening.

References

1. Leder SB, Sasaki CT, Burrell MI. Fiberoptic endoscopic evaluation of dysphagia to identify silent aspiration. Dysphagia. 1998;13:19–21.
2. Baken RJ. Clinical measurement of speech and voice. Boston, MA: College-Hill Press, Div. of Little, Brown, & Co.; 1987.
3. Horner J, Massey EW. Silent aspiration following stroke. Neurology. 1988;38:317–9.
4. Holas MA, DePippo KL, Reding MJ. Aspiration and relative risk of medical complications following stroke. Arch Neurol. 1994;51:1051–3.

5. Leder SB, Espinosa JF. Aspiration risk after acute stroke: comparison of clinical examination and fiberoptic endoscopic evaluation of swallowing. Dysphagia. 2002;17:214–8.

6. Garon BR, Engle M, Ormiston C. Silent aspiration: results of 1,000 videofluoroscopic swallow evaluations. J Neurol Rehabil. 1996;10: 121–6.

7. Smith CH, Logemann JA, Colangelo LA, Rademaker AW, Pauloski BR. Incidence and patient characteristics associated with silent aspiration in the acute care setting. Dysphagia. 1999;14:1–7.

8. Elpern EH, Scott MG, Petro L, Ries MH. Pulmonary aspiration in mechanically ventilated patients with tracheostomies. Chest. 1994;105: 563–6.

9. Leder SB. Incidence and type of aspiration in acute care patients requiring mechanical ventilation via a new tracheotomy. Chest. 2002;122:1721–6.

10. Arvedson J, Rogers B, Buck G, Smart P, Msall M. Silent aspiration prominent in children with dysphagia. Int J Pediatr Ororhinolaryngol. 1994;28:173–81.

11. Linden P, Siebens AA. Dysphagia: predicting laryngeal penetration. Arch Phys Med Rehabil. 1983;64:281–4.

12. Linden P, Kuhlemeier KV, Patterson C. The probability of correctly predicting subglottic penetration from clinical observations. Dysphagia. 1993;8:170–9.

13. Horner J, Massey EW, Riski JE, Lathrop DL, Chase KN. Aspiration following stroke: clinical correlates and outcome. Neurology. 1988;38: 1359–62.

14. Splaingard ML, Hutchins B, Sulton LD, Chaudhuri G. Aspiration in rehabilitation patients: videofluoroscopy vs bedside clinical assessment. Arch Phys Med Rehabil. 1988;69:637–40.

15. Kidd D, Lawson J, Nesbitt R, MacMahon J. Aspiration in acute stroke: a clinical study with videofluoroscopy. Q J Med. 1993;86:825–9.

16. Wakasugi Y, Tohara H, Hattori F, Motohashi Y, Nakane A, Goto S, Ouchi Y, Mikushi S, Takeuchi S, Uematsu H. Screening test for silent aspiration at the bedside. Dysphagia. 2008;23:364–70.

17. Butler SG, Stuart A, Markley L, Rees C. Penetration and aspiration in healthy older adults as assessed during endoscopic evaluation of swallowing. Ann Otol Rhinol Laryngol. 2009;118:190–8.

18. McCullough GH, Rosenbek JC, Wertz RT, Suiter D, McCoy SC. Defining swallowing function by age: promises and pitfalls of pigheonholing. Top Geriatr Rehabil. 2007;23:290–307.

19. Widdecombe JG. Sensory innervation of the lungs and airways. In: Cervero F, Morrison JFB, editors. Progress in brain research. Amsterdam: Elsevier Science Pub; 1986. p. 49–64.

20. Canning BJ, Mazzone SB, Meeker SN, Mori N, Reynolds SM, Undem BJ. Identification of the tracheal and laryngeal afferent neurones mediating cough in anaesthetized guinea-pigs. J Physiol. 2004;557:543–58.

21. McAlexander MA, Myers AC, Undem BJ. Adaptation of guinea-pig vagal airway afferent neurones to mechanical stimulation. J Physiol. 1999;521(Pt.1):239–47.

22. Taylor-Clark T, Undem BJ. Transduction mechanisms in airway sensory nerves. J Appl Physiol. 2006;101:950–9.

23. Sant'Ambrogio FB, Anderson JW, Sant'Ambrogio G. Effect of 1-menthol on laryngeal receptors. J Appl Physiol. 1991;70:788–93.

24. Sant'Ambrogio G, Mathew OP, Sant'Ambrogio FB, Fisher JT. Laryngeal cold receptors. Respir Physiol. 1985;59:35–44.

25. Tsubone H, Sant'Ambrogio G, Anderson JW, Orani GP. Laryngeal afferent activity and reflexes in the guinea pig. Respir Physiol. 1991;86:215–31.

26. Sant'Ambrogio FB, Anderson JW, Sant'Ambrogio G, Mathew OP. Response of laryngeal receptors to water solutions of different osmolality and ionic composition. Respir Med. 1991;85(Suppl):A57–60.

27. Suiter DM, Leder SB. Clinical utility of the 3-ounce water swallow test. Dysphagia. 2008;23:244–50.

28. Suiter DM, Sloggy J, Leder SB. Validation of the yale swallow protocol: a prospective double-blinded videofluoroscopic study. Dysphagia. 2014;29:199–203.

29. Daniels SK, Corey DM, Hadskey LD, Legendre C, Priestly DH, Rosenbek JC, Foundas AL. Mechanism of sequential swallowing during straw drinking in healthy young and older adults. J Speech Hear Lang Res. 2003;47:33–45.

30. Kelly AM, Leslie P, Beale T, Payten C, Drinnan MJ. Fibreoptic endo-scopic evaluation of swallowing and videofluoroscopy: does examination type influence perception of pharyngeal severity? Clin Otolaryngol. 2006;31:425–32.

31. Murguia M, Corey DM, Daniels SK. Comparison of sequential swallow-ing in patients with acute stroke and healthy adults. Arch Phys Med Rehabil. 2009;90:1860–5.

32. Ozaki K, Kagaya H, Yokoyama M, Saitoh E, Okada S, Gonzales-Fernandez M, Palmer JB, Uematsu H. The risk of penetration and aspira-tion during videofluoroscopic examination of swallowing varies depending on food types. Tohoku J Exp Med. 2010;220:41–6.

33. Riccio MM, Kummer W, Bigliari B, Myers B, Undem BJ. Interganglionic segregation of distinct vagal afferent fibre phenotypes in guinea-pig isolated airway. J Physiol. 1996;496:521–30.

34. Verillo RT. Effect of spatial parameters on the vibrotactile threshold. J Exp Psychol. 1966;71:570–5.

35. Green BG, Craig JC. Roles of vibration amplitude and static force in vibrotactile spatial summation. Percept Psychophys. 1974;16:503–7.

36. Gescheider GA, Guclu B, Sexton JL, Karalunas S, Fontana A. Spatial summation in the tactile sensory system: probability summation and neu-ral integration. Somatosens Mot Res. 2005;22:255–68.

37. Green BG, Zaharchuk R. Spatial variation in sensitivity as a factor in measurements of spatial summation of warmth and cold. Somatosens Mot Res. 2001;18:181–90.

38. Nguyen NP, Moltz CC, Frank C, Vos P, Smith HJ, Nguyen PD, Nguyen LM, Dutta S, Lemanski C, Sallah S. Impact of swallowing therapy on aspiration rate following treatment for locally advanced head and neck cancer. Oral Oncol. 2007;43:352–7.
39. Link DT, Willging JP, Miller CK, Cotton RT, Rudolph CD. Pediatric laryngopharyngeal sensory testing during flexible endoscopic evaluation of swallowing: feasible and correlative. Ann Otol Rhinol Laryngol. 2000;109:899–905.
40. Donzelli J, Brady S, Wesling M, Craney M. Predictive value of accumulated oropharyngeal secretions for aspiration during video nasal endoscopic evaluation of swallowing. Ann Otol Rhinol Laryngol. 2003;112: 469–75.
41. Lazarus CL. Effects of chemoradiotherapy on voice and swallowing. Curr Opin Otolaryngol Head Neck Surg. 2009;17:172–8.
42. Leder SB, Ross DA. Investigation of the causal relationship between tracheotomy and aspiration in the acute care setting. Laryngoscope. 2000;110:641–4.
43. Leder SB, Ross DA. Confirmation of no causal relationship between tracheotomy and aspiration status: a direct replication study. Dysphagia. 2010;25:35–9.

Chapter 11
In Support of Use of the Yale Swallow Protocol: Longer-Term (5 Day) Success of Diet Recommendations and Oral Alimentation

Evidence for longer-term success of diet recommendations and oral alimentation after passing the Yale Swallow Protocol has been lacking. Indeed, a search of the literature did not reveal *any* longitudinal data >24 h after passing either a swallow screen or instrumental, FEES or VFSS, dysphagia evaluation. Longitudinal information is needed in order to demonstrate longer-term successful oral alimentation based on passing the Yale Swallow Protocol. The study below answers this important question.

Leder SB, Suiter DM. Five days of successful oral alimentation for hospitalized patients based upon passing the Yale Swallow Protocol. Ann Otol Rhinol Laryngol. (doi: 10.1177/0003489414525589: In Press; 2014). (Used and modified with permission from SAGE Journals.)

Objectives: To determine success of oral alimentation and patient retention rate 1–5 days after passing the Yale Swallow Protocol.

Methods: Participants were 200 consecutive acute care inpatients referred for swallow assessment. Inclusion criteria were adequate cognitive abilities to participate safely, completing an oral mechanism examination, and passing the 3-ounce water swallow challenge. Exclusion criteria were altered mental status, failing the 3-ounce challenge, preadmission dysphagia, head-of-bed restrictions <30°, and a tracheotomy tube. Electronic medical record monitoring post-protocol passing for 1–5 consecutive days determined success of oral alimentation and hospital retention rate.

S.B. Leder and D.M. Suiter, *The Yale Swallow Protocol: An Evidence-Based Approach to Decision Making*, DOI 10.1007/978-3-319-05113-0_11, © Springer International Publishing Switzerland 2014

Results: All patients who remained medically and neurologically stable drank thin liquids and ate successfully during their hospitalization from 1–5 days after passing the protocol. Mean volume of liquid ingested per day was 474.2 cc (sd 435.5 cc). Patient retention declined steadily from day-of-testing ($n=200$) through post-testing day 5 ($n=95$).

Conclusions: Passing the Yale Swallow Protocol allowed for initial determination of aspiration risk followed by successful oral alimentation for 1–5 days in medically and neurologically stable acute care hospitalized patients and without the need for instrumental testing. The decline in patient retention was expected due to increasingly rapid transit through the acute care setting which often renders longer follow-up problematic.

Keywords: Deglutition, Deglutition disorders, Swallow screening, Aspiration risk, Oral alimentation

Introduction

In today's health-care environment optimal patient care, as demonstrated by successful evidence-based interventions, are demanded by both insurers and providers. The 2004–2005 National Hospital Discharge Survey reported that comorbid dysphagia in patients ≥ 75 years of age resulted in a 40 % increase in length-of-stay (2.4 vs. 4.0 days), an additional 223,027 hospitalization days per year, and at a staggering cost of $547,307,964 [1]. Therefore, avoidance of prandial pulmonary aspiration as a cause of nosocomial infection is an important goal for all acute care hospitalized patients deemed at risk for aspiration.

Referral for a swallow evaluation must result in use of either a validated screen or instrumental test with the dual capabilities to reliably determine aspiration risk and appropriately recommend oral alimentation. Surprisingly, no studies, to date, reported >24 h of follow-up for oral feeding status based upon passing either a swallow screen or an instrumental dysphagia evaluation. Not surprisingly, the realities of the acute care setting have limited the ability to track and collect longitudinal data due to acute medical or neurological status changes, rapid discharge from inpatient to home or extended care facilities, and billing regulations that preclude follow-up after a negative test result.

Three studies from the acute care setting reported on ≤24 h of success for oral alimentation recommendations. Twenty-four hours after passing the Yale Swallow Protocol [2] and remaining medically and neurologically stable all intensive care unit [3], acute stroke [4], and general hospital [5] patients were both eating and drinking successfully. Although supportive of short-term benefits a longer follow-up period is needed to either demonstrate continued success of oral alimentation or record potential overt aspiration events later in the patient's clinical course. It is important to note that the focus of the present investigation was not to determine adequacy of oral nutrition and hydration in hospitalized patients. The purposes of the present study were to investigate longer-term success of oral alimentation recommendations and hospital retention rate for up to 5 days after passing the Yale Swallow Protocol.

Each patient referred for a swallow assessment was administered, when deemed appropriate (See flow diagram Fig. 8.1), the Yale Swallow Protocol by an experienced speech-language pathologist. Inclusion criteria were adequate cognitive abilities to participate safely in the protocol [6], completion of an oral mechanism examination [7], and passing the 3-ounce water swallow challenge [8]. Exclusion criteria were severely altered mental status precluding safe participation in the protocol, failing the 3-ounce water swallow challenge, a current modified consistency diet due to a preexisting dysphagia, head-of-bed restrictions <30º, and presence of a tracheotomy tube [3–5]. Referred patients who failed the protocol were not included.

Yale Swallow Protocol

The Yale Swallow Protocol incorporated, validated, and generalized use of the 3-ounce water swallow challenge component, originally used in isolation with a small ($n=44$) cohort of stroke patients in the rehabilitation setting [9], to a large ($n=3,000$) and heterogeneous

(14 diagnostic categories) sample of hospitalized individuals [8]. Subsequent double-blinded objective testing with fiberoptic endoscopic evaluation of swallowing (FEES) [7, 10] and videofluoroscopic swallow studies (VFSS) [11] confirmed that all participants who passed the protocol also did not aspirate, i.e., sensitivity of 100 % and negative predictive value of 100 %.

The Yale Swallow Protocol has three components: (1) a 3-ounce water swallow challenge [8]; (2) a brief cognitive screen comprised of three orientation questions, i.e., What is your name? Where are you right now? What year is it? And three single-step directions, i.e., Open your mouth, Stick out your tongue, Smile [6]; and (3) an oral mechanism examination that assessed labial closure, lingual range of motion, and facial symmetry (smile/pucker) [7] with the latter two again using a large and heterogeneous sample of hospitalized individuals ($n = 4,102$).

It is important to note that results of the brief cognitive screen [6] and oral mechanism examination [7] provide the clinician information only on odds of aspiration risk with the 3-ounce water swallow challenge and should not necessarily be used as exclusionary criteria for screening. The reason is that some patients will pass the 3-ounce challenge despite altered mental status and impaired oral mechanism functioning.

Each participant was administered the Yale Swallow Protocol by experienced speech-language pathologists with over 10 years of protocol administration. Passing required uninterrupted drinking (assisted or independent) of 3 ounces of water from a cup or with a straw and with no overt signs of aspiration risk, i.e., cough. Failure was inability to drink the entire amount, interrupted drinking, or coughing during or immediately after drinking. When passed, an oral diet was recommended based on combined results of the cognitive screen, oral mechanism examination, and dentition status. For example, edentulous patients were usually recommended a liquid and puree consistency diet while dentate patients a soft or regular diet. When failed, the options are continued nil-per-os status with repeat screening in 24 h, FEES done immediately at bedside, or VFSS within 24 h.

Standard oral intake as routinely entered by nursing in each patient's electronic medical record allowed for retrieval of the total volume of liquid ingested for days 1–5. Nurses were blinded to the oral intake purpose of the study. A preexisting protocol

TABLE 11.1.   Participant demographic (used with permission from SAGE Journals: Leder SB, Suiter DM. Five days of successful oral alimentation for hospitalized patients based upon passing the Yale Swallow Protocol. Ann Otol Rhinol Laryngol. doi: 10.1177/0003489414525589: In Press: 2014).

Gender	n	Mean age (year)	Age range (year)
Male	129	67.8	18–98
Female	71	68.8	13–98

TABLE 11.2.   Participant diagnostic categories (used with permission from SAGE Journals: Leder SB, Suiter DM. Five days of successful oral alimentation for hospitalized patients based upon passing the Yale Swallow Protocol. Ann Otol Rhinol Laryngol. doi: 10.1177/0003489414525589: In Press: 2014).

Diagnostic category	Number of participants
General medicine	53
Pulmonary	29
Neurosurgery	20
Other neurologic[a]	19
Head and neck cancer	17
Right stroke	15
Cardiothoracic surgery	12
Left stroke	11
Cancer	9
Orthopedic surgery	9
Brainstem stroke	5
Esophageal surgery	1
Total	200

[a]Parkinson's disease, seizure disorder, degenerative, dementia

directed nursing to discontinue the oral diet and re-consult speech-language pathology if overt signs of prandial aspiration occurred, e.g., coughing or choking. Patient retention rate required passing the protocol and then with no overt signs of aspiration risk at mealtimes, stable medical and neurological status, and not discharged from the hospital between day-of-testing and day 5.

A consecutively referred sample (August 15, 2011 to December 01, 2011) of 200 inpatients from a large, urban, acute care, teaching hospital participated. All patients were referred for a swallow assessment by a physician, physician assistant, or licensed independent provider.

Table 11.1 shows participant demographics including age and gender. Table 11.2 shows admitting diagnostic categories.

TABLE 11.3.   Volume (in cc) of liquid ingested per day after passing the Yale Swallow Protocol (used with permission from SAGE Journals: Leder SB, Suiter DM. Five days of successful oral alimentation for hospitalized patients based upon passing the Yale Swallow Protocol. Ann Otol Rhinol Laryngol. doi: 10.1177/0003489414525589: In Press: 2014).

Day	Volume of liquid ingested	Mean standard deviation
1	355.6	398.0
2	519.2	458.0
3	485.1	403.6
4	509.1	424.0
5	501.9	496.9
Total	474.2	435.5

TABLE 11.4.   Nutrition and hydration delivery routes (used with permission from SAGE Journals: Leder SB, Suiter DM. Five days of successful oral alimentation for hospitalized patients based upon passing the Yale Swallow Protocol. Ann Otol Rhinol Laryngol. doi: 10.1177/0003489414525589: In Press: 2014).

Delivery routes	n	%
Nil per os	95	47.5
Nasogastric/Nasojejunal tube	69	34.5
Per os	19	9.5
Gastrostomy/Jejunostomy tube	11	5.5
Total parenteral nutrition	6	3.0
Total	200	100

Table 11.3 shows results of oral intake data as entered by nursing into the electronic medical record. Neither the speech-language pathology nor nursing services identified any patient as exhibiting overt signs of aspiration risk at mealtimes. All patients who passed the protocol and maintained a stable medical and neurological status while hospitalized drank and ate successfully without overt signs of aspiration risk up to and including post-testing day 5. Mean volume of liquid ingested per day for the entire sample was 474.2 cc (sd 435.5 cc). The recommended diets spanned thin liquids with puree, soft solid, or regular solid consistency foods dependent upon cognition and dentition status.

Table 11.4 shows nutrition and hydration delivery routes. A total of 181 (90.5 %) patients had a nil-per-os order and were receiving

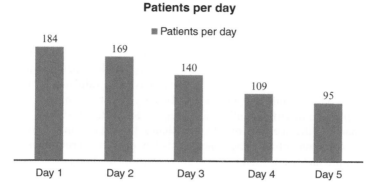

FIG. 11.1.   Patient retention rate per day of hospitalization (used with permission from SAGE Journals: Leder SB, Suiter DM. Five days of successful oral alimentation for hospitalized patients based upon passing the Yale Swallow Protocol. Ann Otol Rhinol Laryngol.; doi: 10.1177/0003489414525589: In Press: 2014).

enteral or parenteral nutrition concomitant with referral for a swallowing evaluation. Nineteen (9.5 %) patients were ordered an oral diet in addition to being referred for a swallow evaluation.

Figure 11.1 shows that patient retention decreased steadily from day-of-testing ($n=200$; 100 %) through post-testing day 5 ($n=95$; 48 %). The majority of patients ($n=60$) were discharged on post-testing days 3 ($n=29$) and 4 ($n=31$). Sixteen (8 %) patients were discharged from the hospital either on day-of-testing or post-testing day 1. Eight (4 %) patients were made nil per os due to inability to maintain inclusion criteria, i.e., worsening medical or neurological conditions. Four (2 %) patients did not eat or drink anything, only taking sips of liquid, despite passing the protocol, during the 5-day follow-up period but rather relied totally on a nasogastric or nasojejunal ($n=3$) or gastrostomy ($n=1$) feeding tube for delivery of nutrition and hydration.

For the first time, long-term success of oral alimentation after swallowing testing has been documented. Passing the Yale Swallow Protocol [2] allowed for initial determination of aspiration risk followed by up to 5 days of successful oral alimentation in hospitalized patients.

These long-term results corroborated short-term (<24 h) eating and drinking success with intensive care unit [3], acute stroke [4], and general hospital [5] patients. The Yale Swallow Protocol meets all criteria necessary for a successful screening tool, i.e., simple and inexpensive to administer [12], quick to perform and interpret [13], reliable, accurate, and timely [14], validated for use with other health-care professionals, e.g., registered nurses [2], applicable to virtually all patients regardless of diagnosis [8], and spanning the age spectrum from pediatric [15] to geriatric [16].

The protocol is strengthened by its key operating criteria and a unique factor not found in any other instrument. The key criteria include determination of aspiration risk with both a high sensitivity of 96.5 % and a high negative predictive value of 97.9 % [8], and, since silent aspiration is volume dependent, a low false negative rate of <2.0 % [17]. The unique factor is a priori knowledge of successful swallowing with thin liquid, puree, and solid food consistencies because the 3-ounce challenge [8] was performed in conjunction with and corroborated by double-blinded testing with both FEES [7, 10] and VFSS [11]. This allows for specific diet recommendations to be made safely, confidently, and in a timely fashion without the need for instrumental dysphagia diagnostic testing [8] in virtually all hospitalized patients who are deemed potential candidates for oral alimentation [3–5, 8].

The findings of the present study are corroborated by previous research. Specifically, the mean amount of liquid ingested orally per day during this study (474.2 cc) was in agreement with short-term (<24 h) amount of liquid ingested by studies which focused on intensive care unit (360 cc) [3], acute stroke (385 cc) [4], and general hospital (340 cc) [5] patients. The approximate 120 cc increase can be attributed to the benefits afforded by longer-term follow-up which allowed for health improvement leading to enhanced oral alimentation. Importantly, the present study's population sample (Tables 11.1 and 11.2) with respect to age ranges, gender differences of more males than females, and admitting diagnostic categories was consistent with a much larger ($n = 4{,}038$) epidemiologic study on aging and dysphagia in the acute care hospitalized population [16] thereby increasing reliability and generalizability of results.

A total of 69 (34.5 %) patients successfully supplemented oral nutrition and hydration with enteral alimentation via nasogastric or nasojejunal tubes (Table 11.4). Previous research demonstrated that the presence of a nasal feeding tube, regardless of age, diagnostic category, or tube diameter, did not increase incidence of aspiration for either liquid or puree food consistencies [18, 19]. Therefore, a swallowing evaluation can be performed with a nasal feeding tube in place and there is no contraindication, as the present study has demonstrated, to continuing supplemental enteral nasal tube feeding until prandial nutrition and hydration are adequate.

Despite passing the Yale Swallow Protocol a total of four (2 %) patients relied on enteral tube feedings thereby choosing not to eat and taking only sips of liquid. This is not unexpected in the acute care setting. It is important to note that passing the protocol permits safe oral alimentation but cannot mandate compliance. A lack of appetite and subsequent desire to eat per os occurs due to feeling unwell or satiety from tube feedings. These patients should be referred to a registered dietitian in order to adjust tube feedings, e.g., reducing flow rate or cycling to night, with the goal of maintaining adequate nutrition and hydration concomitant with increasing oral alimentation.

Although the present study documented success of long-term oral alimentation, it must be emphasized that swallowing assessment provides only a snapshot-in-time of a patient's swallowing abilities and neither subjective nor objective testing can guarantee continued successful swallowing behavior. The clinician must be aware that a negative test allows for safe eating and drinking only as long as the patient remains stable. Therefore, caregivers must remain vigilant to signs of aspiration risk, e.g., coughing at mealtimes, altered mental status, or symptoms of upper respiratory infection, and recommend timely reevaluation.

Conclusions

In conclusion, all patients who maintained the inclusion criteria were successfully drinking thin liquids and eating 1–5 days after passing the Yale Swallow Protocol. Mean volume of liquid ingested per day for the entire sample was 474.2 cc (sd 435.5 cc).

Patient retention decreased steadily from day-of-testing ($n=200$) through post-testing day 5 ($n=95$). This was expected due to increasingly rapid transit through the acute care setting which often renders longer follow-up problematic. For the first time, longer-term success of oral alimentation after swallowing testing has been documented. Passing the Yale Swallow Protocol allowed for initial determination of aspiration risk followed by longer-term success of up to 5 days of oral alimentation in acute care hospitalized patients and without the need for instrumental testing.

References

1. Altman KW, Yu G-P, Schaefer SD. Consequence of dysphagia in the hospitalized patient. Arch Otolaryngol Head Neck Surg. 2010; 136:784–9.
2. Warner HL, Suiter DM, Nystrom K, Poskus, K, Leder SB. Comparing accuracy of the Yale Swallow Protocol when administered by registered nurses and speech-language pathologists. J Clin Nursing. (In Press) doi: 10.1111/jocn.12340.
3. Leder SB, Suiter DM, Warner HL, Kaplan LJ. Initiating safe oral feeding in critically ill intensive care and step-down unit patients based on passing a 3-ounce (90 milliliters) water swallow challenge. J Trauma. 2011;70:1203–7.
4. Leder SB, Suiter DM, Warner HL, Acton LM, Swainson BA. Success of recommending oral diets in acute stroke patients based on a 90-cc water swallow challenge protocol. Top Stroke Rehabil. 2012;9:40–4.
5. Leder SB, Suiter DM, Warner HL, Acton LM, Siegel MD. Safe initiation of oral diets in hospitalized patients based on passing a 3-ounce (90 cc) water swallow challenge protocol. Q J Med. 2012;105:257–63.
6. Leder SB, Suiter DM, Lisitano HL. Answering orientation questions and following single step verbal commands: effect on aspiration status. Dysphagia. 2009;24:290–5.
7. Leder SB, Suiter DM, Murray J, Rademaker AW. Can an oral mechanism examination contribute to the assessment of odds of aspiration? Dysphagia. 2013;28:370–4.
8. Suiter DM, Leder SB. Clinical utility of the 3 ounce water swallow test. Dysphagia. 2008;23:244–50.
9. DePippo KL, Holas MA, Reding MJ. Validation of the 3-oz water swallow test for aspiration following stroke. Arch Neurol. 1992;49: 1259–61.
10. Leder SB, Judson BL, Sliwinski E, Madson L. Promoting safe swallowing when puree is swallowed without aspiration but thin liquid is aspirated: Nectar is enough. Dysphagia. 2013;28:58–62.

11. Suiter DM, Sloggy J, Leder SB. Validation of the Yale Swallow Protocol: A prospective double-blinded videofluoroscopic study. Dysphagia. 2014;29:199–203.
12. Heffner JE. Swallowing complications after endotracheal extubation. Chest. 2010;137:509–10.
13. Cochrane AL, Holland WW. Validation of screening procedures. Br Med Bull. 1971;27:3–8.
14. Kertscher B, Speyer R, Palmieri M, Plant C. Bedside screening to detect oropharyngeal dysphagia in patients with neurological disorders: An updated systematic review Dysphagia (In Press). doi: 10.1007/s00455-013-9490-9
15. Suiter DM, Leder SB, Karas DE. The 3-ounce (90 cc) water swallow challenge: a screening test for children with suspected oropharyngeal dysphagia. Otolaryngol Head Neck Surg. 2009;140:187–90.
16. Leder SB, Suiter DM. An epidemiologic study on aging and dysphagia in the acute care hospitalized population: 2000–2007. Gerontology. 2009;55:714–8.
17. Leder SB, Suiter DM, Green BG. Silent aspiration risk is volume dependent. Dysphagia. 2011;26:304–9.
18. Leder SB, Suiter DM. Effect of nasogastric tubes on incidence of aspiration. Arch Phys Med Rehabil. 2008;89:648–51.
19. Fattal M, Suiter DM, Warner HL, Leder SB. Effect of presence/absence of a nasogastric tube in the same person on incidence of aspiration. Otolaryngol Head Neck Surg. 2011;145:796–800.

Chapter 12
Final Thoughts

Objectives: To demonstrate the reliability, validity, and generalizability of the Yale Swallow Protocol as a swallow screen for determining both aspiration risk as well as safe and appropriate oral diet recommendations.

Methods: A total of over 5,000 patients, from 14 different diagnostic categories, representative of all medical and surgical hospital specialties, and spanning the age spectrum from pediatric to geriatric participated. FEES and VFSS were the criterion standards confirming aspiration risk.

Results: The Yale Swallow Protocol has achieved two important goals. Its high sensitivity of 96.5 %, high negative predictive value of 97.9 %, and low <2 % false negative rate make it an excellent swallow screen for determination of aspiration risk status. After passing and remaining medically and neurologically stable pediatric, trauma, acute stroke, and general hospital patients demonstrated 100 % successful eating and drinking for up to 5 days making the protocol a clinically useful and efficient screen.

Conclusions: The Yale Swallow Protocol is a reliable, validated, and generalizable swallow screen. When administered and interpreted by a trained specialist the protocol may be adopted as a standard clinical assessment tool for both determination of potential aspiration risk and to make recommendations for initiating specific oral diets without the need for further instrumental testing.

S.B. Leder and D.M. Suiter, *The Yale Swallow Protocol: An Evidence-Based Approach to Decision Making*, DOI 10.1007/978-3-319-05113-0_12, © Springer International Publishing Switzerland 2014

Keywords: Deglutition, Deglutition disorders, Swallow screen, Oral alimentation

Final Thoughts

We have shown that the foundation, development, and implementation of the Yale Swallow Protocol are all grounded in an evidence-based approach to decision making for evaluation of potential aspiration risk status and determination of specific oral diet recommendations. All seminal and supportive data have been published in peer-reviewed journals. No findings or recommendations have been conjectures unsupported by facts. Our patient population sample was large and heterogeneous; specifically: over 5,000 patients; from 14 different diagnostic categories; representative of every medical and surgical intensive care unit and general hospital service; and spanning the age spectrum from pediatric to geriatric participated in the various published studies that are integral to the protocol's success. Additionally, it was shown that not only speech-language pathologists but registered nurses (and we hope that future research includes other health-care professionals) can administer and interpret the protocol accurately and correctly.

One true measure of any swallow screen depends on its simplicity. The Yale Swallow Protocol adheres to the principle of Occam's Razor or The Least Complicated Explanation. It is comprised of a brief cognitive evaluation, an oral mechanism examination, and a 3-ounce water swallow challenge. These three components are readily comprehensible to and easily employed by all health-care professionals. There is no long questionnaire, no subjective assessment of variables such as voice quality or cough strength, and no use of an unproven swallowing task.

The protocol, however, does need to be administered in a precise manner every time. It is useful to think of the administering clinician as akin to a baseball umpire who calls the play by the rule book and has no vested interest in whether the player (patient) is safe (passes) or out (fails). Similarly, the clinician like the umpire must not be influenced by the fans (family), e.g., "I hope my child/

father/mother passes.", personal emotion, e.g., "I hope my patient passes.", or preconceived thinking, e.g., "My patient should fail so no need to administer the protocol." The bottom line is you cannot know the outcome without playing the game or in our scenario administering and interpreting the protocol correctly.

Additionally, for a screening tool to be successful it must be able to be used by different clinical specialists and with virtually all at-risk individuals. (The only exception is when a patient has a tracheotomy tube.) The question that always needs to be asked is: Are the results and recommendations working to benefit the patient? With respect to the dual purposes of the Yale Swallow Protocol, it not only reliably identifies patients who are an aspiration risk but also is efficient regarding making appropriate decisions concerning specific diet recommendations. That is, when passed patients can be ordered the appropriate oral diet without the need for further instrumental testing. One purpose without the other is not helpful to the clinician, patient care, efficiency, or cost containment.

Since 2008 the Yale Swallow Protocol has been administered to more than 15,000 acute care patients at both Yale-New Haven Hospital and VAMC Memphis. Its use has changed our clinical practice for the better. To reiterate, patients identified as being an aspiration risk and subsequently referred for a swallow assessment are, when deemed appropriate, first administered the protocol. When the protocol is passed patients are recommended an oral diet and oral medications without undue delay. The diet is usually regular if dentition or dentures are adequate or puree if dentition is inadequate and dentures are ill-fitting or not available. When the protocol is failed appropriate referral to speech-language pathology is made for either instrumental testing or rescreening in 24 h. Continuity of care has been demonstrated as both short-term 1-day and longer-term 5-day follow-up studies have corroborated the efficacy and success of eating and drinking after passing the protocol.

Future research concerning use of the Yale Swallow Protocol in the rehabilitation setting and for an even longer period of time than 5 days is of great interest. Also, investigating generalizability of use of the Yale Swallow Protocol by health-care professionals other than registered nurses such as physicians and physician assistants is an important goal. Questions never stop being asked because the answers are so interesting.

The development and implementation of the Yale Swallow Protocol have been our personal Homeric Odyssey since 1999. Although it took Ulysses (only) 10 years to return home from Troy our clinical care journey took 5 years longer but we have finally reached our metaphorical Ithaca with publication of this book. (This geographical coincidence must not be lost on the reader as SBL earned a Bachelor of Science degree in speech-language pathology from Ithaca College which is in, of course, Ithaca (!) New York.)

The Yale Swallow Protocol has not only changed our professional lives but also enabled us to deliver evidence-based state-of-the-art clinical care to our patients—and both for the better. We trust you agree with us and will use the Yale Swallow Protocol to the benefit of both yourselves and your patients. We thank you but most important of all your patients will thank you.

Best,
Steven B. Leder
Debra M. Suiter

Chapter 13
Yale Swallow Protocol Administration Forms

Administration Form 1.

Yale Swallow Protocol

Step 1: Exclusion Criteria

__ **Protocol Deferred: NO risk factors for aspiration.**

Protocol deferred if any YES answer to the following criteria

Yes	No	
__	__	Unable to remain alert for testing
__	__	No thin liquids due to preexisting dysphagia
__	__	Head-of-Bed restricted to <30°
__	__	Tracheotomy tube present
__	__	Nil-per-os order for medical/surgical reason

If a patient's clinical status changes resulting in a new risk for aspiration re-administer protocol before oral intake of food or medicine.

S.B. Leder and D.M. Suiter, *The Yale Swallow Protocol: An Evidence-Based Approach to Decision Making*, DOI 10.1007/978-3-319-05113-0_13, © Springer International Publishing Switzerland 2014

Administration Form 2.*

Yale Swallow Protocol

Step 2: Administration Instructions

**Perform protocol if patient is an aspiration risk and
ALL Step 1 boxes are checked NO**

- **Brief Cognitive Screen[a]**: __ What is your name?   __ Open your mouth

    __ Where are you right now? __ Stick out your tongue

    __ What year is it?   __ Smile

- **Oral-Mechanism Examination[b]**: __ Labial closure

    __ Lingual range of motion

    __ Facial symmetry (smile/pucker)

- **3-Ounce Water Swallow Challenge[c]**:

- Sit patient upright at 80-90° (or as high as tolerated >30°)

- Ask patient to drink the entire 3 ounces (90cc) of water from a cup or with a straw, in sequential swallows, and slow and steady but without stopping
  (Note: Cup or straw can be held by staff or patient)

- Assess patient for coughing or choking during or immediately after completion of drinking

  [a,b] Information from the brief cognitive screen and oral mechanism examination
      provide information only on odds of aspiration risk with the 3-ounce water
      swallow challenge and should not be used as exclusionary criteria for screening.
  [c] It is permissible to repeat the 3-ounce water swallow challenge if it is thought
      the patient may pass with a second attempt.

Administration Form 3.*

Yale Swallow Protocol

Step 3: Pass/Fail Criteria

Results and Recommendations

___   **PASS: Successful uninterrupted drinking of all 3 ounces of water without overt signs of aspiration (coughing/choking) either during or immediately after completion.**

- If patient passes, collaborate with MD/PA/LIP to order appropriate oral diet.

- If adequate dentition order a soft solid consistency or regular consistency diet.

- If inadequate dentition or edentulous order a liquid and puree diet.

- Consult with speech-language pathologist for other diet modifications.

___   **FAIL: Inability to drink the entire 3 ounces in sequential swallows due to interrupted drinking (stopping/starting) or patient exhibits overt signs of aspiration (coughing/choking) either during or immediately after completion.**

- If patient fails, keep nil per os (including medications) and request the MD/PA/LIP to order a consult for an instrumental swallowing evaluation by speech-language pathology.

  OR

- Continue nil-per-os status and re-administer the protocol in 24 hours if patient shows clinical improvement.

- If patient fails again request the MD/PA/LIP to order a consult for an instrumental swallowing evaluation by speech-language pathology.

* S.B. Leder and D.M. Suiter, *The Yale Swallow Protocol: An Evidence-Based Approach to Decision Making*, © Springer International Publishing Switzerland 2014

Index

A

Acton, L. M., 84
Acute care
  hospitalize patients, 92, 93, 134
  settings, 94, 101, 123, 134, 141
Acute stroke patients,
  generalization to,
    84–88, 93–95
Administration
  forms, 149–151
  protocol, 106–108
Adult acute care population,
  generalization to, 76–77
Aging
  epidemiologic study
    demographic information, 9
    diagnostic categories, 9, 10
    non-oral feeding, 13
    oral feeding status, 11, 12
    population data, 10, 11
  of general population, 14
Airway maintenance, tracheotomy
  tube for, 32–33, 94
American Speech Language and
  Hearing Association
  (ASHA), 3
Aspiration
  prandial pulmonary, 90, 134
  risk for potential, 90
Aspiration pneumonia, 21
  prandial, 113, 116

Aspiration risk
  case-finding approach, 20–21
  CSE *vs.*, 3–5
  determination, 4, 99–100, 145–148
    non-swallowing variables, 31
  dysphagia *vs.*, 2–3
  in geriatric population, 6–7
  identification, 123, 125
  screening tests for, 19–20, 73
    determination, 22
  status, 73
  swallow screening for
    goals, 37
    potential, 112
    reliability testing, 40–41
    research questions and
      answers, 37–39, 41–46
Aspiration status, cognitive
  examination
  clinical importance, 60–61
  FEES
    outcomes, 56
    testing, 54–56
  liquid aspiration, 56–57
    commands follow, 59
  oral intake, 58
    commands follow, 59–60
  Pearson's chi-square analysis, 59
  puree aspiration, 57
    commands follow, 59
  swallow screening protocol, 53

C

Chemo-radiation therapy, 94, 122, 128
Clinical or bedside swallow
        examination (CSE)
    oral diet recommendations, 4–5
    vs. screening for aspiration risk,
        3–5
Cognition, 106, 138
The Comprehensive Level of
        Consciousness Scale, 54
Cost-effective screening test, 113

D

Deglutition disorders, 83
DePippo, K. L., 5
Dysphagia
    vs. aspiration risk, 2–3
    epidemiologic study
        demographic information, 9
        diagnostic categories, 9, 10
        non-oral feeding, 13
        oral feeding status, 11, 12
        population data, 10, 11
    evaluation, 61
    incidence of, 14
    referral rates for, 10, 12
    tablet swallowing, 102

F

Fiberoptic endoscopic evaluation
        of swallowing (FEES),
        2, 4, 13
    advantage, 31
    diet recommendations, 42–44
    examination, oral mechanism
        diagnostic categories, 64
        labial closure/facial
            symmetry, 66–68
        lingual range of motion,
            66–68
        participant demographics, 64
        reliability testing, 65–66
    instrumental testing with, 73, 74
    liquid aspiration, 41–42

    outcomes, 56
    protocol, 38, 108
        silent aspiration, 124
    reliability testing, 40–41
    results, 46–47
    test, 54, 56, 75

G

General hospital patients,
        generalization to, 88–95
Geriatric population, aspiration risk
        in, 6–7
Geriatrics, swallowing problems in,
        6–7
Green, B. G., 120

H

Health-care professionals
    for aspiration risk, 14
    Yale Swallow Protocol
        implementation, 111–117
Heffner, J. E., 30

K

Kaplan, L. J., 77
Karas, D. E., 72

L

Laryngeal desensitization, 33
    silent aspiration, 94, 128
Laryngeal mechanoreceptors, 126
Leder, S. B., 4, 7, 51, 61, 72, 77,
        79, 84, 100, 111, 120,
        124, 133
Likelihood ratios (LR)
    advantage, 26
    definition, 26

M

Mechanoreceptors, laryngeal, 126
Murray, J., 61

N
Nystrom, K., 111

O
Oral alimentation, 4, 7
    negative test, 101
    potential candidates for, 5
    resumption of, 13
        promote safe, 14, 15
    success for, 109
Oral alimentation, for hospitalize
            patients
    aspiration risk determination, 140
    long-term, 139, 141
    oral intake, 136–138
    prandial pulmonary aspiration, 134
    retention rate, 139
    swallow assessment, 135
    Yale Swallow Protocol, 135
        components, 136
        screening tool, 140
Oral diets, 99–101
    ongoing monitoring, 101–102
    tablet swallowing, 102
Oral mechanism FEES examination
    diagnostic categories, 64
    labial closure/facial symmetry,
            66–68
    lingual range of motion, 66–68
    participant demographics, 64
    reliability testing, 65–66

P
Pediatric population, generalization
            to, 72–76, 93–95
Poskus, K., 111
Prandial aspiration pneumonia, 113,
            116
Prandial pulmonary aspiration, 90, 134

R
Rademaker, A. W., 61
Razor, Occam, 146

Registered nurses (RNs), 113–116
Reliability testing, 40–41, 65–66
    intra-and inter-rater, 124–125

S
Screening test, swallow, 2
    accuracy of, 23–25
    for aspiration risk, 19–20, 73
        determination, 22
    assumptions, 21
    criteria for, 4
    disadvantage of, 24, 25
    false positive/negative rates, 25
    likelihood ratios, 26
    positive/negative predictive
            values, 25
    sensitivity, 24
    specificity, 24–25
    3-ounce water, 5–6, 13
Screening tool, 4, 7, 14, 22, 111,
            128, 140, 147
    accuracy of, 23
    criteria for, 72
Silent aspiration
    chemo-radiation therapy, 128
    definition, 119
    FEES protocol, 124
    intra-and inter-rater reliability
            test, 124–125
    laryngeal desensitization, 94, 128
    laryngeal mechanoreceptors, 126
    rate, 126
    risk
        identification, 123, 125
        volume-dependent
                determination, 126
    spatial summation, 127
    swallow screen determination,
            120
Stroke patients, generalization to,
            84–88, 93–95
Suiter, D. M., 4, 7, 51, 61, 72, 77,
            79, 84, 100, 111, 120,
            124, 133
Swainson, B. A., 84

Swallowing disorders, 7, 14, 21–22, 76, 85
Swallowing problems, 22, 71, 73, 94, 101
    in geriatrics, 6–7
    identification of, 113, 117
Swallowing task, 120, 128, 146
    aspiration risk status, 83
    importance of, 6
Swallow screening
    for aspiration risk
        goals, 37
        potential, 112
        reliability testing, 40–41
        research questions and answers, 37–39, 41–46
    clinical judgment, importance, 33
    in clinical practice, guidelines, 4
    cognitive screen, 30
    criteria
        for failure, 30, 31
        for successful, 29
    definition, 2
    determination, silent aspiration, 120
    nasogastric and orogastric feeding tube, 32
    non-swallowing stimuli, 31
    protocol, 53
    Yale Swallow Protocol as, 145–148
Swallow screening test, 2
    accuracy of, 23–25
    for aspiration risk, 19–20, 73
        determination, 22
    assumptions, 21
    criteria for, 4
    disadvantage of, 24, 25
    false positive/negative rates, 25
    likelihood ratios, 26
    positive/negative predictive values, 25
    sensitivity, 24

    specificity, 24–25
    3-ounce water, 5–6, 13

T
3-ounce water swallow challenge
    diet recommendations, 42–44
        water test, 45
    generalizability of, 75
    and liquid aspiration, 41–42
        water test, 43
    synthesize and discuss results, 46–47
3-ounce water swallow test, 5–6, 13
Tracheotomy tube, for airway maintenance, 32–33, 94
Trauma patients, generalization to, 93–95
    ICU/SDU patient, 78–82
    oral diet recommendations, 82–83

V
Videofluoroscopic swallowing study (VFSS), 2, 4, 13, 81
    instrumental test with, 73, 74
    irradiation exposure with, 75
    protocol, 109

W
Warner, H. L., 51, 77, 84, 111

Y
Yale Swallow Protocol
    administration, 106–108
        forms, 149–151
    failure, 108–109
    generalization
        adult acute care population, 76–77

general hospital patients, 88–95
pediatric population, 72–76,
    93–95
stroke patients, 84–88, 93–95
trauma patients, 77–84, 93–95

implementation, 111–117
oral diets, 99–101
    ongoing monitoring, 101–102
    tablet swallowing, 102
as swallow screen, 145–148

Lightning Source UK Ltd.
Milton Keynes UK
UKOW06f2108310316

271250UK00013B/43/P